APPLIED HUMAN NUTRITION
For Food Scientists and Home Economists

ELLIS HORWOOD SERIES IN FOOD SCIENCE AND TECHNOLOGY

Editor-in-Chief: I. D. MORTON, Professor and formerly Head of Department of Food and Nutritional Science, King's College, University of London.
Series Editors: D. H. WATSON, Ministry of Agriculture, Fisheries and Food; and
M. J. LEWIS, Department of Food Science and Technology, University of Reading

Fats for the Future   R.C. Cambie
Food Handbook   C.M.E. Catsberg & G.J.M. Kempen-van Dommelen
Principles and Applications of Gas Chromatography in Food Analysis   M.H. Gordon
Vitamins and Minerals in Health and Nutrition   M. Tolonen

Forthcoming titles
Food Biochemistry   C. Alais & G. Linden
Traditional Fermented Foods   M.Z. Ali & R.K. Robinson
Food Microbiology, Volumes 1 & 2   C.M. Bourgeois, J.F. Mescle & J. Zucca
Determination of Veterinary Residues in Food   N.T. Crosby & C.M. Clark
Food Container Corrosion   D.R. Davis & A.V. Johnston
Technology of Meat and Meat Products   J. P. Girard
Dairy Technology   A. Grandison, M.J. Lewis, R.A. Wilbey & R.K. Robinson
Separation Processes: Principles and Applications   A. Grandison & M.J. Lewis
Microbiology of Chilled and Frozen Foods   W.F. Harrigan
Nitrate and Nitrites in Food and Water   M.J. Hill
Modern Food Processing   J. Lamb
Food Technology Data   M.J. Lewis
Technology of Biscuits, Crackers and Cookies, 2nd Edition   D.J.R. Manley
Second European Conference on Food Science and Technology   I.D. Morton
Modified Atmosphere Packaging of Food   B. Ooraikul
Food, Volumes 1 & 2   P. Patel
Feta and Related Cheeses   R.K. Robinson
Handbook of Edible Gums   K.R. Stauffer
Applied Human Nutrition: For Food Scientists and Home Economists   A.F. Walker
Natural Toxicants in Food   D.H. Watson

APPLIED HUMAN NUTRITION
For Food Scientists
and Home Economists

Editor

ANN F. WALKER B.Sc., D.T.A., M.Sc., Ph.D.
Lecturer in Human Nutrition
Department of Food Science and Technology
University of Reading

ELLIS HORWOOD
NEW YORK LONDON TORONTO SYDNEY TOKYO SINGAPORE

First published in 1990 by
ELLIS HORWOOD LIMITED
Market Cross House, Cooper Street,
Chichester, West Sussex, PO19 1EB, England

A division of
Simon & Schuster International Group
A Paramount Communications Company

Printed and bound in Great Britain
by Hartnolls, Bodmin, Cornwall

Exclusive distribution by Van Nostrand Reinhold/AVI London:
Australia and New Zealand:
CHAPMAN AND HALL AUSTRALIA
Box 4725, 480 La Trobe Steet, Melbourne 3001, Victoria, Australia
Canada:
NELSON CANADA
1120 Birchmount Road, Scarborough, Ontario, Canada, M1K 5G4
Europe, Middle East and Africa:
VAN NOSTRAND REINHOLD/AVI LONDON
2–6 Boundary Row, London SE1 8HN, England
North America:
VAN NOSTRAND REINHOLD/AVI NEW YORK
115 Fifth Avenue, 4th Floor, New York, New York 10003, USA
Rest of the world:
THOMSON INTERNATIONAL PUBLISHING
10 Davis Drive, Belmont, California 94002, USA

British Library Cataloguing in Publication Data

Applied human nutrition.
1. Man. Nutrition
I. Walker, Ann F.
613.2
ISBN 0–7476–0049–X

Library of Congress Cataloging-in-Publication Data

Applied human nutrition for food scientists and home economists / editor, Ann F. Walker.
p. cm. — (Ellis Horwood series in food science and technology)
Includes bibliographical references.
ISBN 0–7476–0049–X
1. Nutrition. 2. Nutrition disorders. 3. Diet. I. Walker, Ann (Ann F.) II. Series.
[DNLM: 1. Diet. 2. Food-Processing Industry. 3. Nutrition. 4. Nutrition Disorders. QU 145
A6515]
TX353.A67   1989
363.8–dc20
DNLM/DLC
for Library of Congress   90–4270
                                                                                 CIP

List of Contributors

Professor Arnold E. Bender
(formerly, Professor of Nutrition, King's College, University of London)
2 Willow Vale, Fetcham, Leatherhead, Surrey KT22 9TE.

Professor Michael I. Gurr
Nutrition Consultant
Milk Marketing Board, Thames Ditton, Surrey KT7 0EL.

Dr Anthony R. Leeds MB ChB
Lecturer in Nutrition
Department of Food and Nutritional Sciences, King's College, University of London, Kensington Campus, Campden Hill Rd, London W8 7AH.

Dr David P. Richardson
Manager, Scientific Services
Nestle Company Ltd, St George's House, Croydon, Surrey CR9 1NR.

Dr Hugh M. Sinclair DM FRCP (deceased, June 1990)
Director, International Nutrition Foundation
High Street, Sutton Courtenay, Abingdon, Oxfordshire, OX14 4AW.

Dr Ann F. Walker
Lecturer in Nutrition,
Department of Food Science and Technology, University of Reading PO Box 226, Reading, RG6 2AP.

Table of Contents

Table of Contents

Table of Contents

Foreword

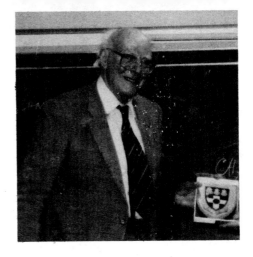

This book serves both as a guide on applied human nutrition and as a memorial to Dr Hugh Sinclair (picture above), who died just before its completion. (Aspects of the life and work of Hugh Sinclair are told in the fine booklet published by the McCarrison Society* in June this year.)

With his work at Oxford, no one had done more to keep alive the scientific basis of human nutrition during the decades following World War II. Medical historians will record with incredulity how, in 1946 the Ministry of Health, the Medical Research Council and University of Oxford could have come to the conclusion that everything was already known about human nutrition, and that monies for nutrition research should be diverted to studies on feeding animals! The offer to fund a Wellcome Institute of Human Nutrition at Oxford was actually declined! Hugh and I served together on the 1950 BMA (British Medical Association) Nutrition Committee which reviewed the war-time diet and its effects on the health of the nation. Its recommendation to keep human nutrition under continuing review was also rejected!

Paradoxically, it may have been the success of the Ministry of Food during the dark war years which may have blinded those in the corridors of power to the need for further research in human nutrition. It has proved to be a most expensive mistake in terms of loss of health for the nation. We won the battle for health during the war and then lost it in the postwar decades.

During the War and immediately afterwards (1941–1946), the mortality at all ages in Great Britain dipped sharply, continuing to fall and finishing well below the expected level based on the steady decline since the previous century. These war years were the only years during the twentieth century when most people of all ages had a near optimal intake of essential nutrients, thanks to the universal use of the 85% extraction National Loaf and to the remarkably well-orchestrated campaign on the Home Front to promote the consumption of 'protective' foods. Although only 27 of the nearly 50 essential nutrients had been identified by then, the choice of foods recommended, and the many hints given on preserving their nutritional value, contributed advice that could well have been written today. With more whole foods, more pulses, more home-grown fruit and vegetables and more variety, health was maintained. (Fortunately, enough imported food escaped the submarines to provide sufficient calories, but it was a near thing!) Petrol rationing, more physical exercise, the will to win, the moderation of energy intake by the consumption of less fat and sugar all made contributions, but the main support for our defences against infection would have come from our intake of nutrients.

This timely publication brings together not only Hugh Sinclair's contributions on nutritional history and essential fatty acids, but also our present knowledge about the nutrients that the consumer needs in order to maintain vitality, virility and freedom from illness. It is a positive approach, which we need again if the rising generation is to avoid the current epidemic of obesity, coronary heart disease, cancer and various other 'diseases of affluence', and to keep diabetes under control. The present-day advice on the prevention of illness has become far too negative, with so much emphasis on just reducing fats and sugars. The real need is to concentrate positively on the nutrients that we require to maintain cellular metabolism and health, including the vitamins, trace elements, essential fatty acids and antioxidants, that are endangered by the storage, refining and processing of foods. We need to define clearly their important food sources, such as the fibre-rich foods, whole grain foods, pulses, nuts, fruit, vegetables and fish.

Dr Ann Walker has brought together the essential knowledge for Food Scientists and Home Economists to advise the public positively on food and health during the Nineties and into the next century.

Sir Francis Avery Jones
Chairman, Council of Management
International Nutrition Foundation
Sutton Courtenay, Oxfordshire.

July 1990

*The McCarrison Society, c/o Eileen Fletcher, 25 Tamar Way, Woose Hill, Wokingham, Berkshire RG11 9UB.

Preface

This book was written with final-year food science and Home Economics undergraduate and postgraduate students particulary in mind, although others with a sound background in the sciences may also find it useful reference text. While the approach assumes a knowledge of basic nutrition, the focus of the book is on those aspects of nutrition at the interface of nutrition and food science, which impinge on food production and consumer concerns. Information on some of the subjects covered is only available elsewhere in detailed reviews or in other scientific literature, which may not be easily accessible to students. For this reason, food technologists working in the food industry may also derive benefit from reading it. In addition, since the book addresses aspects of nutrition both in health and disease, dietitians, nurses and medical students may find it a useful resource text, when dealing with queries raised by the public.

Nutrition is being increasingly recognized as fundamental to good human health: a principle to which all nutritionists are committed. All of the six nutritionists who have contributed chapters to this book have many years of experience of working in their particular branches of the subject. Each has his or her own views of controversial areas, which I have made no attempt to alter or influence.

The aim of the book has been to provide an accessible approach, without too many detailed references, for students for whom nutrition is only part of their course. However, suggestions for further reading are given with each chapter. Although the approach to the subject is appropriate for a student text, the various arguments that go to make up the contentious issues in nutrition have not been avoided. For example, the validity of the Recommended Daily Amounts of nutrients in predicting the adequacy of the diet of the individual has been thoroughly discussed by Professor Bender (Chapter 1).

The objectives of human nutrition are health and wellbeing, both nebulous concepts which it is not possible to measure directly. By comparison, in farm animal nutrition, objectives such as weight gain make the assessment of good nutrition easy and this often explains why the nutrient requirements of animals are known more precisely than they are for humans. In addition, there are the problems of the ethics of human experimentation, which are discussed by Dr Sinclair (Chapter 3). Therefore, published data derived from human experimentation should be carefully scrutinized to determine the exact protocol under which it was conducted, as different conditions may lead to different results. Failure to do so may give rise to contradictory interpretation of experimental data which could account for the all-to-often poor image of nutritionists in the mind of the public as those offering conflicting advice.

Apart from my gratitude to the other authors involved in this book, there are other acknowledgements that I wish to make. I particulary thank Dr Alan Lakin, my husband,

Preface

for his support, encouragement and his conviction of the importance of nutrition to health. Also my thanks are due to the Photographic Department of the University of Reading for preparing the plates for Chapter 3. I am also indebted to my many students of the Department of Food Science and Technology, who have given me enthusiatic feedback on the nutrition course which led to the development of this book, to Dr Mike Lewis for suggesting that these lectures might be made available to a wider audience, and finally to the University of Reading, for providing the ethos that has stimulated and facilitated the work.

May 1990

Ann F. Walker

Abbreviations

AP	As purchased
BDA	British Diabetics Association
BHA	Butylated hydroxy anisole
BHT	Butylated hydroxy toluene
BMI	Body mass index
CHD	Coronary heart disease
CHO	Carbohydrate
COMA	Committee on Medical Aspects of Food Policy, Ministry of Agriculture, Fisheries and Food, UK.
DHA	Docosahexaenoic acid
DHSS	Department of Health and Social Security (UK Government)
EC	European Community
EFA	Essential fatty acids
EP	Edible portion
EPA	Eicosapentaenoic acid
FAC	Food Advisory Committee of MAFF (see below)
FAO	Food and Agriculture Organization of the United Nations
GIP	Gastric inhibitory peptide
HDL	High density lipoproteins
HPLC	High pressure liiquid chromatography
IDDM	Insulin-dependent diabetes mellitus
IgA	Immunoglobulin A
IgG	Immunoglobulin G
IQ	Intelligence quotient
LACOTS	Local Authorities Committee on Trading Standards (UK)
LDL	Low density lipoproteins
MAFF	Ministry of Agriculture, Fisheries and Food (UK)
MOD	Mature-onset diabetes
NACNE	National Advisory Council for Nutrition Education, UK
NAD	Nicotinamide adenine dinucleotide
NFS	National Food Survey (UK)
NIDDM	Non-insulin-dependent diabetes mellitus
P/S ratio	Polyunsaturated fatty acids to saturated fatty acids ratio
PUFA	Polyunsaturated fatty acids (polyunsaturates)

Abbreviations

RDA	Recommended Daily Amount (UK), Recommened Dietary Allowance (USA)
SMA	Scientific milk adaptation
TB	Tuberculosis
TG	Triglyceride(s), now known as triacylglycerol(s)
VLCD	Very low calorie diet(s)
VLDL	Very low density lipoproteins

1

Eating for health

Arnold Bender

Introduction

This chapter deals broadly with the subject of nutrition and briefly covers topics which are dealt with in more detail in later chapters. Many people these days talk about 'healthy eating', but this is an ambiguous phrase which is not easy to interpret and poses the question of what is 'unhealthy eating'. I much prefer to talk about 'an adequate diet' or 'sensible eating'.

One 'half' of nutrition is an attempt to answer the question 'Are we adequately fed?' and I emphazise this, as we are rather obsessed these days with diseases of affluence such as coronary heart disease, diverticular disease, obesity, and forms of cancer which may be linked to diet, and tend to forget that we need all the nutrients in adequate amounts to grow, develop and resist infection and disease.

How does one know what a good or adequate diet is? We read criticisms in newspapers that fast foods and convenience foods are 'bad' and that baked beans are dreadful because they contain sugar. It is important in nutrition to think quantitatively. When a journalist says that there is sugar in baked beans, this is true, as it comprises about 3 – 4% of the weight. However, the average consumption of baked beans in the UK is about 100 g per head per week, which would yield only about 3–4 g of sugar per week from this source.

THE 'FIRST HALF' OF NUTRITION

It is not easy to answer the question, 'What is a good or adequate diet?' Much knowledge exists on the nutrients required by human beings. We know that we need 13 vitamins, 20 mineral salts, amino acids, certain essential fatty acids and, of course, adequate energy. It is the 'how much?' of each of these nutrients that is more doubtful. This question is only partly addressed by published tables called **Recommended Daily Amounts (RDA)** of nutrients, which are derived from measurements of nutrient requirements, with an extra amount added for good measure. There are three main approaches for measuring these requirements:

(1) *Observation of population groups (Epidemiology)*. Consider, for example, vitamin B_1 (thiamin), a lack of which may result in the clinical deficiency state called beri-beri. The incidence of beri-beri is high in some areas of the world, but does not occur in other regions. Such observations can be correlated with thiamin intake, leading to the conclusion that 0.4 mg of thiamin is required per 1000 non-fat calories to prevent beri-beri. (NB: Thiamin is required for the breakdown of carbohydrates.)

Unfortunately, this approach is applicable to very few nutrients, because for most of them it usually takes months on a deficient diet before clinical signs of deficiency show. The method can be applied to neither proteins nor minerals, and to only a few vitamins. Thus, for example, this approach is not appropriate for vitamin A, as this is stored in the body to a considerable extent.

(2) *Animal experimentation*: In this approach, animals are made deficient by feeding a diet low in or lacking the nutrient in question. They are then fed diets containing the nutrient at various levels to determine the level which will cure the deficiency. Alternatively, diets containing varying levels of the nutrient can be fed to groups of animals and the level required to prevent deficiency occurring noted. This is a **prophylactic** (preventive), rather than a **therapeutic** approach.

One of the main problems with using animals as models for human nutrition is converting the requirements of other species to those of human beings. Another problem is the selection of appropriate parameters on which to base nutrient requirement. This can be on the basis of body weight, food consumed, surface area, or lean active body mass. Only if the precise function of the nutrient under study is known, can the right parameters be selected.

(3) *Experimentation on human subjects*: Data derived from human experiments are scarce, as such experiments are tedious, costly and extremely difficult to perform. Experiments of this nature cannot be conducted for more than a few weeks at a time, because of loss of volunteers' motivation.

Therefore, data from human experiments are far from complete. We have data from 20-year-old subjects because many investigations have been carried out on university students. There is also data for babies. Nutrient requirements for babies are derived differently from those for adults, being based on human milk intake, rather than on observing, for example, the first signs of deficiency, a method which is considered unethical when applied to babies as they cannot volunteer for experiments. However, very little is known about the nutrient requirements of other human groups. Therefore, between infancy and 20 years, we interpolate, and for older groups we extrapolate.

With the limitations of the methods described, and the paucity of the data, figures for the *physiological requirements* of nutrients for different groups can only be approximate. Thus, these are figures, which, in the opinion of experts and in the light of contemporary knowledge, best represent the requirements for a particular nutrient. The *mean* nutrient requirement of a selected human group is then converted into the RDA (Recommended Daily Amount) for most nutrients (apart from energy) by adding to it two standard deviations (see below). This intake will take care of the needs of those in the selected human group, even with above-average requirements. As RDAs are calculated on a population basis, they apply to population groups and not to individuals. Thus an individual cannot be assessed as malnourished on the basis of a finding of a nutrient intake below the RDA.

Nutrient intake levels: High enough to prevent deficiency or to saturate tissue?
In setting RDA's a particular thorny problems is to decide what nutrient status is being used as the objective. The various levels are shown in Figure 1.1.

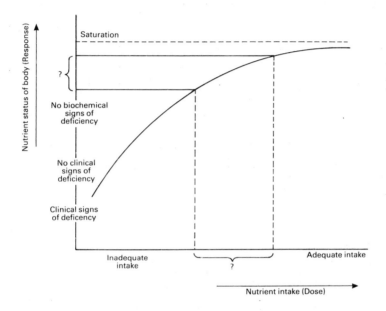

Fig. 1.1 — Dose/response relationship for a nutrient.

The intake of a nutrient is plotted along the horizontal axis, while on the vertical axis are the clinical and biochemical signs of nutrient status. Obviously, at a low level of intake, clinical signs of deficiency occur, giving rise, for example, to characteristic signs, such as rickets, scurvy or beri-beri (deficiencies in vitamins D, C and thiamin, respectively). Clearly, this level of intake would be inadequate. With a higher intake of the nutrient, the clinical signs will disappear. But the question remains, 'Is that enough?': is it satisfactory to say that if there are no clinical signs, then intake of that nutrient is adequate?

This question is not easily answered, and the answer may differ depending on the nutrient. One complication is that there can be more than one sign of deficiency of the same nutrient. For example, scurvy is prevented with 10 mg of vitamin C per day, but wound healing is delayed until one provides 20 mg per day. With high doses, one can reach a level at which there are no measurable biochemical signs (e.g. optimal level of enzyme function). At higher levels of intake, one will eventually reach a point of tissue saturation. Saturation implies that an intake above this level (certainly of the water soluble vitamins) would not be utilised, but would be excreted.

The question remains 'Is one 'better off' in health if the tissues are saturated with nutrients?' Tests for tissue nutrient status of any particular nutrient usually show that most of us are not 'saturated', even though we show no signs of deficiency that can be measured (in other words, higher levels could be achieved in tissues). For most nutrients, there are wide differences between nutrient levels which appear to be clinically adequate and those which would saturate tissues, so there is scope for differences of opinion between these two levels on appropriate intakes for health.

Having decided the criteria for determining an adequate nutrient level, selecting an RDA for a particular population group is complicated by individual variation in requirements of nutrients, which can be very large. From any group of, say, 20 volunteers, the measured requirements can vary by as much as 100%: i.e. the lowest requirement will be half that at the top end of the scale.

Figure 1.2 shows the usual basis for setting an RDA for a nutrient. It shows the idealized distribution curve for the measured requirements of a nutrient for a particular human group. The mid-point represents the mean requirement for the group, and obviously, many people require this amount. A smaller number have requirements above average and a very small number have very high requirements. Similarly, at the other end of the distribution curve, a small number of people require less than average, and (so far as we know) there are a very small number of people with very low requirements.

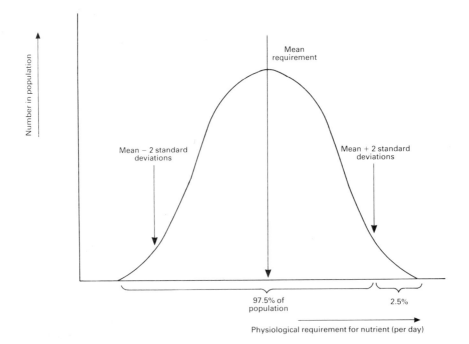

Fig. 1.2 — The basis for setting the RDA (Recommended Daily Amount) for a nutrient for a specified human group.

When using RDAs, it must always be borne in mind that data such as those presented in Figure 1.2 are based on relatively small numbers of subjects. In addition, the distribution curve is assumed to be 'normal' (or Gaussian). This is in keeping with the medical concept of normality, in which any measurable parameter of a human group (e.g. blood glucose level) is deemed to provide a normal distribution. This may or may not be the case in reality, and it is rare in nutrition to have so much data that the hypothesis can be properly tested.

In Figure 1.2 the mean value plus or minus two standard deviations (SD) includes 95% of the population. Hence, if RDAs are set at the mean + 2 SD they cover the needs of the 'greater part' of the population (97.5%). A statement to this effect is found in most RDA Tables. Theoretically, 2.5% of the requirement of any human group will be higher than the RDA.

From the shape of the curves for most nutrients (except protein), 2 SD would result in a difference of 20% of the mean value (for protein the value is 30%). Thus intakes of less than 20% below the mean, i.e. 40% below RDA, would, theoretically, at least, be inadequate for nearly everyone. It is important to remember that RDAs apply to *population groups* and not to *individuals*, but if the intake of an individual is less than 60% of RDA for long periods, then he or she is likely to become deficient. A dietary intake of a nutrient greater than 80% of the RDA can be regarded as a rough estimate of what we mean by an adequate diet (for most people).

Table 1.1 — European RDAs for selected Nutrients for an adult male

	Protein	Vitamins					
		A	E	B$_1$	B$_2$	B$_6$	C
	(g)	(µg)	(mg)	(mg)	(mg)	(mg)	(mg)
France	81	1000	15	1.5	1.8	2.2	80
Germany	63	900	12	1.6	2.0	1.8	75
Italy	64	750	—	1.1	1.5	—	45
Netherlands	70	450	—	1.1	1.6	—	50
Spain	54	750	—	1.1	1.6	—	45
UK	69 (10%E)	750	—	1.1	1.5	—	30
Scandinavia	10–15%E	1000	—	1.4	1.5	2.2	60

B$_1$, thiamin; B$_2$, riboflavin; B$_6$, pyridoxine; %E, protein energy as a percentage of total dietary energy; RDA, Recommended Daily Amount; µg, micrograms; mg, milligrams.

Table 1.1 lists the RDAs of some nutrients of six European countries plus Scandinavia, and shows some intriguing differences. In the UK the RDA for protein is a flat rate of 10% of the energy of the diet, rather than an absolute figure, while in other countries the RDA is based on requirement figures derived from nitrogen balance studies. This difference in method of calculating the RDA leads to a very wide range of recommendations for protein — from 54 to 81 g per day. The vitamin A RDA also shows a wide (twofold) range.

Four countries and Scandinavia concluded that there is not enough evidence on which to base a figure for vitamin E and (excepting Scandinavia) vitamin B_6, while the other countries conclude that there is — again, this is a matter of consensus opinion. The RDAs for B_1 (thiamin), for which we ought to have fairly precise figures (because of the ease of obtaining data for this nutrient using the epidemiological approach — see above), nevertheless still vary by 50%. The values for vitamin C show nearly a threefold range!

So, despite the available experimental evidence, much still depends on the opinions of the specific committee deliberating *at that time*. When using RDAs for labelling food products, a single value is needed, rather than a different one for each human group. Even more care should therefore be used in interpreting RDAs used on food labels. RDAs for use in labelling throughout the European Community have been produced by *Codex Alimentarius* (Table 1.2). It is likely that each European country will continue to have its own RDAs for *health purposes* for specific human groups.

Table 1.2 — Vitamin and mineral RDAs for food labelling in the European Community

Vitamin A µg	1000
Vitamin D µg	5
Vitamin E µg	10
Vitamin C mg	60
Thiamin mg	1.4
Riboflavin mg	1.6
Niacin mg	18
Vitamin B_6 mg	2
Folacin µg	400
Vitamin B_{12} µg	3
Biotin mg	0.15
Pantothenic acid mg	6
Calcium mg	800
Phosphorous mg	800
Iron mg	12
Magnesium mg	300
Zinc mg	15
Iodine µg	150

The committee assigned the task of revising the 1979 UK RDA tables should report by 1990–91. It is likely that many more nutrients will be included than in the previous report, including the vitamins, B_6, E and K, and the minerals, zinc and iodine. This is not necessarily because there is better information than in 1979, but because of the demand for RDAs in making nutritional claims. Currently, since there are no British RDAs for a number of nutrients, manufacturers use those published in the USA and this has caused some confusion.

In attempting to assess whether or not a diet is adequate, apart from the problems of defining requirements,¡ there are the additional problems of measuring nutrient intake. We could measure food intake including total energy by weighed dietary survey over a specified time period (typically seven days). If the person is not gaining or losing weight, then their intake of energy must fulfil their requirements. On this basis, the range in adult human energy intakes is very large with the highest showing a three-fold or four-fold difference from the lowest.

People at the lower end of the range can live well on 1200 kcals per day, while those at the high end of the range need over 4000 kcals per day. Those on low energy intakes, if they are eating the same diet as those with high intakes, would also be getting about a third of the protein, minerals and vitamins compared to those at the top of the range. However, it is not known if they require only a third of these other nutrients. They certainly require only a third of the B vitamins if they are taking in a third of the carbohydrate, as the B vitamins are used in the metabolism of the carbohydrate and, therefore, the requirement for these depends on the intake of carbohydrate. However, as far as vitamins A and C are concerned, it may be that requirements of these are related to body size rather than energy expenditure. The problem is that we do not know whether people who need a third of the energy of other people, also require only a third of other nutrients.

With so much imponderability regarding the nutrient requirements of an individual, we lack a truly scientific approach when dealing with the question of whether an individual is adequately fed. Under these circumstances it is tempting to suggest that he or she might take a nutrient supplement and just observe whether of not any benefit accrues.

Assessing Nutritional Status
In industrialized countries, we rarely observe any clinical signs of nutrient deficiency. Even when there are mild signs of what appears to be a deficiency, it is difficult to decide whether such changes are due to nutritional deficiency or to one of several other causes, let alone to decide which nutrient is the problem. For example, a red tongue can be a sign of riboflavin deficiency, but there can be several other causes. Only in severe and chronic cases of nutrient deficiency are the clinical signs characteristic and even then, not always.

If there are suggestive clinical signs, then biochemical examination is called for. For example, tissue levels of NAD (nicotinamide adenine dinucleotide) are determined if niacin deficiency is indicated. Although such biochemical tests are more objective, the problem is the lack of any standard level with which to compare the individual's measure. So-called 'normal values' are based on the medical concept of normality (see above). However, a level below 'normal values' may be quite normal for some individuals.

If a person is showing some clinical or biochemical sign of nutrient deficiency, the obvious next step is to examine the diet. This might show that the intake of a specific nutrient is below the RDA. However, some individuals can live on diets 60% below the RDA and still be adequately fed. A final step would then be to supply the suspect nutrient. If the disorder then cleared up this would be a clear indication that the person had been deficient in that nutrient.

Thus, the three methods available for determining whether an individual is adequately fed, i.e. clinical, biochemical and dietary assessment, can, in the final analysis, only be used as indicators of inadequate nutrition, and the proof of correct diagnosis would be if the disorder disappeared when the nutrient suspected of being deficient was supplied.

In the well-nourished western world a slight deficiency may presumably occur without any clinical signs. If a nutritional supplement is provided many individuals will 'improve', as they will on an inert supplement. This is the placebo effect, which has been shown in clinical trials to benefit (improve the 'condition' of) 30% of subjects.

The discussion above still raises the question of whether or not the average person would be better off taking nutrient supplements. By definition, if you have an adequate diet you will have full body *nutrient stores* and you will be clinically in good health (Figure 1.3).

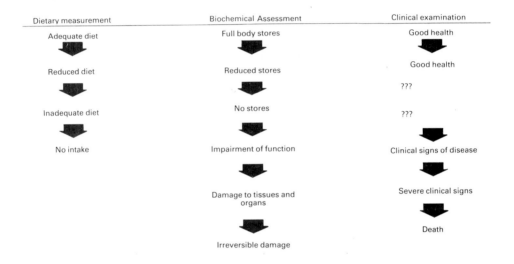

Fig. 1.3 — Assessment of human nutritional status.

If intake of a nutrient is reduced, the first result will be to reduce body stores. That will not matter for nutrients like vitamin A, since most people have about two year's supply in their livers. However, if the vitamin A-deficient diet continues, eventually the individual will be left with no stores.

The adverse consequences of 'no stores' is debatable, particularly if the nutrient is supplied regularly in adequate amounts. The problem arises when the individual had an inadequate store *and* the intake of the nutrient becomes inadequate. The first effect is biochemical, i.e. an impairment of function, such as a reduced level of a coenzyme (biochemical lesion). It is only when deficiency is more severe that damage to tissues occurs and clinical signs appear. Early on, such clinical signs are mild and reversible, but, if the nutrient deficiency continues, irreversible damage occurs, leading to severe clinical signs and, eventually, to death.

To summarize. In the western world, clinical signs of nutrient deficiency would not be expected, so how do we know if someone is adequately nourished or would be any 'better' if they took a supplement? The short answer is that we don't know. All we can say is that one should improve the diet as much as possible, making sure that it is varied and that the processing (including domestic cooking) of the food is not so severe or prolonged that vitamins are extensively damaged. Having said that, there is no way of being sure that a particular individual would not benefit from nutrient supplementation.

Balance of the major sources of energy in the diet

One important point to bear in mind when considering the balance of the major sources of energy in the diet is the other nutrients that are contained in these sources. In the UK, about 40% of the energy of our diet comes from fat, 15% from sugar and, on average, 5% from alcohol. So, for the average person, two thirds of the dietary energy comes from 'empty calories' (meaning energy sources which are devoid of or low in nutrients). A person consuming such a diet would, therefore, rely on one third of his or her food to supply *all* the nutrients.

Reducing the content of empty calories in the diet would automatically increase the content of those sources of energy that carry nutrients with them, thus improving the overall quality of the diet. For example, eating a diet containing less sugar and more bread would give extra minerals, protein and vitamins from the bread that could not be supplied by the sugar. Fats are not entirely 'empty calories' as most contain essential fatty acids and some carry vitamins, although the amounts vary (refined oils contain very low levels).

A varied diet will supply all the nutrients required for health, even if only by chance. If the diet is restricted then there is much less chance of this: hence nutritional advice is to eat a *varied diet*.

Are dietary supplements beneficial?

Apart from medical cases and people living on bizarre diets, nobody is sufficiently poorly fed in the UK to show clinical signs of deficiency, but would they be any better off if given supplements? Because of the placebo effect it is difficult, almost impossible, to answer this question.

The difficulties of interpreting the beneficial effects of supplementation, if any, are shown in the following example. It was reported in the *Lancet* (Benton and Roberts, 1988) that giving children vitamin and mineral supplements improved their IQ (ability to learn). Following media coverage, vitamin tablet sales rocketed. However, interpretation of this study is hampered by lack of baseline (initial) vitamin intakes. The experiment was repeated by another research team on larger numbers of children, who found no effect of supplementation on IQ (Naismith *et al.*, 1988).

THE 'SECOND HALF' OF NUTRITION

Trends in Longevity

Despite our modern life style and the recent publicity, not merely about food poisoning, but concerning the consumption of high-fat diets or convenience and fast foods, and about young people who do not eat traditional meals, people are living longer. One cynical view might be that people who are in their 80s today have lived through two world wars and the great Spanish influenza epidemic of 1918 and have, therefore, been naturally selected for their toughness. If this is true, then perhaps in a few years time we might find that the length of life is declining. Certainly, people in industrialized countries such as the UK have suffered increasingly in recent decades from the 'diseases of affluence', including coronary heart disease. These diseases, according to expert committees who draw up **guidelines on diet**, are more associated with the levels of the major sources of energy in the diet than the levels of particular nutrients. Guidelines on diet (Table 1.3) include recommendations to decrease the fat and sugar content of the diet, and have modified the nutritionists' maxim 'eat a little of everything' to 'eat a little of everything and not too much of any one thing'.

Table 1.3 — Summary of dietary guidelines of NACNE (1983) and COMA (1984)

(1) Lose excess weight

(2) Reduce fat intake to about 30% of dietary energy.

(3) If necessary for taste and texture, replace saturate fats with polyunsaturates, but do not add these to the diets as an extra.

(4) Reduce intake of sugar.

(5) Replace fats and sugar with starchy foods — preferably whole grain.

(6) Increase intake of dietary fibre — fruits, vegetables and whole grain cereals.

(7) Reduce intake of salt.

(8) Keep alcohol intake to moderate amounts.

Coronary heart disease (CHD)
Much attention has been paid to CHD since it is the cause of about one third of the male deaths and a high proportion of female deaths in the UK. In epidemiological studies, a strong correlation has been found between blood cholesterol levels and the incidence of and the mortality from CHD.

The main factors affecting blood cholesterol are heredity, maleness, lack of exercise and smoking, but the principal dietary factor is saturated fat. The association is not all that strong with saturated fat (the strength of the association is shown in Fig. 1.4 by the thickness of the arrow). It is considered by some authorities that a reduction in blood cholesterol levels will reduce the hazard of CHD — but even this has not been unequivocally proven.

High blood cholesterol levels can be lowered by dietary means, by restricting the intake of saturated fat, and by the use of drugs. Increasing the dietary fibre content of the diet has much less effect, although experimentally, the soluble fibres, as found in oats, have been shown to be effective.

Risk factors in CHD
Total dietary fat and saturated fats in particular, have been widely publicized as major risk factors in CHD. However, many other factors have also been implicated: Hopkins

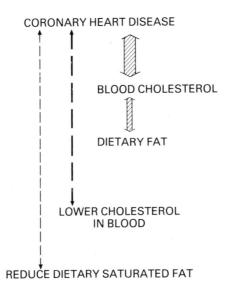

CORONARY HEART DISEASE

BLOOD CHOLESTEROL

DIETARY FAT

LOWER CHOLESTEROL
IN BLOOD

REDUCE DIETARY SATURATED FAT

Fig. 1.4 — Relative strengths of major risk factors and preventative measures in the aetiology
of coronary heart disease.

and Williams (1981) listed 246 such factors. To qualify for inclusion in the list, their
criterion was that the factor had been shown to be a risk for CHD in at least one
published paper in a properly refereed journal. Since that time, at least six more factors
have been added.

Risk factors range from blood parameters, physical and physiological signs, to diet
and even rate of growth of beard in men and deep religious conviction (the last is a
protective factor). It is likely that there is no one causative factor, but a large range,
which is usually referred to as lifestyle, together with hereditary features.

The influential COMA Report (DHSS, 1984) on *Diet and cardiovascular disease*
gave recommendations for modifying diet to reduce the incidence of CHD. It was written
with much greater caution than has subsequently been publicized in the media. The
following are quoted from the conclusions:

(1) Comparison between countries of *epidemiological* data shows a strong positive
correlation between saturated fat intake and coronary heart disease. (However,
within countries there is no convincing evidence of such a relationship.)

(2) Within any one of several countries epidemiological data show a strong positive relation between total plasma cholesterol and heart disease.

(3) Clinical trials show that dietary saturated fatty acids increase plasma cholesterol level.

The Report continues:

> There is emerging evidence that reduction of plasma cholesterol may be associated with slower progression of artherosclerotic lesions.

And for those identified as at risk of CHD:-

> 'the incidence of CHD has been reduced by decreasing plasma cholesterol by diet and or drugs.'

The Report points out that the 'final link' establishing a causal relationship directly between the intake of saturated fat and the incidence of CHD has not been established. It is doubtful, because of the magnitude of the experimental procedure, that proof will ever be forthcoming on this point, as this would require that people be kept for very long periods of their life on strictly controlled diets, which is impractical. Despite the limitations of the evidence, the COMA Report concludes:

> There is sufficient consistency in this evidence to make it more likely than not that the incidence of CHD will be reduced by decreasing the intake of saturated fatty acids and total fat. The evidence falls short of proof.

There is a great gap between the cautious statements of the medical experts and nutritionists and the headlines which are getting through to the public. Unfortunately it is the headlines which are remembered.

Other 'diseases of affluence', including cancer

A similar problem arises with other diseases of affluence. It is suggested, and again, the evidence is epidemiological rather than experimental, that certain forms of cancer may be caused or associated with a high-fat diet. One of these is cancer of the breast. There is also a suggestion that a high blood carotene level is protective against cancer of the lung. In an attempt to find a link between the incidence of lung cancer and carotene intake, the first studies were *retrospective* epidemiological studies (where people with cancer were identified and questioned on their past eating habits). Retrospective studies are fraught with difficulty and are very imprecise. People do not remember what they ate and they certainly cannot be very quantitative. So retrospective studies are simply an indication that there might be a link, and cannot be taken as causative.

Prospective studies are more reliable. For a study of this type, large numbers of people are kept under observation for several years and their food intake measured at intervals. This information is then correlated with the appearance of the disease in question. This approach in costly in time and human resources. One approach is to take blood samples from all subjects at the beginning of the study and store them frozen; then, when the disease state is eventually diagnosed, to analyse the blood and compare it with the matched controls taken at the same time. This approach, while yielding more precise data, measures the factor in the blood and not in the diet. In the case of the possible protective effect of carotene on the development of lung cancer, there are at least two very large-scale trials currently being carried. One is a five-year intervention trial on 29,000 people in Finland. Half the subjects are given carotene capsules, while the other half are receiving placebo. The results are awaited with interest.

Dietary guidelines
Despite the lack of proof of the link between diet and diseases of affluence, dietary goals or guidelines have been drawn up in many countries throughout the world (Table 1.3).

There is no doubt that the goals appear straightforward and simple, but the relations between dietary changes and disease are complex and subject to debate.

Ideal body weight
It is accepted that obesity is a health hazard, but there is no ideal body weight for a person of a given height. Recent height/weight tables give an acceptable range (see Chapter 6): 10% above the upper end of this range is termed overweight and 20% is termed obesity. While there does not appear to be a direct relation between CHD and overweight, overweight exacerbates other disorders, such as hypertension (high blood pressure), which have a more direct relation to CHD.

While a small degree of excess weight may have no clinical result this might well be an early stage of weight gain which will lead to obesity. Since prevention of obesity is easier to achieve than later weight loss, a slow increase of weight should be regarded as an early warning.

Dietary fat
Fat intake in countries with a high incidence of CHD is around 40% of total energy intake, although this same intake figure is common in Mediterranean countries such as Greece, where the incidence of CHD is low. It is suggested that the difference lies in the type of fat — largely olive oil (high in monounsaturated fatty acids) in Mediterranean countries, compared with much more saturated fats in northern Europe. There is a consensus of opinion that a more appropriate figure for fat intake would be 30–35% of the diet, but that figure has no firm basis. The incidence of CHD in various countries has been rising and falling over the years without any known change in total fat intake.

Nevertheless, fat intake, especially of saturated fats, has been shown in clinical trials to raise blood cholesterol level, which is a known risk factor for CHD. However, there is still much debate as to whether reducing the levels of blood cholesterol, either by diet or by drug treatment, confers any benefit.

Compliance with dietary guidelines is fraught with difficulty. It is clearly difficult for anyone, even a nutritionist, to simply and routinely monitor his or her fat intake. In addition, the concept of 35% of dietary energy as fat is incomprehensible to the layman, so the advice must be simply to reduce the fat wherever possible, irrespective of any knowledge of the individual's actual intake.

Polyunsaturated fatty acids
There is some confusion between different authorities about adding polyunsaturates to the diet. The COMA Report clearly states that the aim is to reduce total fat, and that

polyunsaturates should not be added to the diet, but used to replace saturates where appropriate.

There is evidence that a high intake of polyunsaturates can lead to the formation of free radicals, with detrimental effects, unless intakes of *antioxidant nutrients* (see Chapter 7) are at appropriate levels.

Dietary cholesterol

American and British official opinion on the importance of dietary cholesterol intake in influencing blood cholesterol levels differs considerably. The US Senate Report (McGovern 1977) states that the average US intake of 600 mg of cholesterol a day is too high and should be reduced to about 300 mg. The COMA Report states that the UK intake of 350–450 mg a day is not excessive and that evidence for an influence of this level of intake on blood cholesterol is inconclusive.

Several trials have shown no increase in blood cholesterol with an increase in dietary cholesterol; others have shown a small increase when the diet was also rich in fat. In practice, reducing the intake of fat will automatically reduce the intake of cholesterol.

Sugar

NACNE guidelines (1983) suggested that the sugar in the diet be reduced to 10% of total dietary energy from present levels (about 15–20%). While there is little firm evidence for a role of high sugar intake in the aetiology (cause) of disease, other than in dental caries, any reduction in sugar intake tends to be automatically balanced by an increased intake of other foods — most of which will supply nutrients in addition to the energy.

Dietary fibre

NACNE (1983) suggested that the diet of an adult should contain on average 30 g of dietary fibre per day rather than 20 g per day as it does as present. However, even if an increase is desirable, there is no basis for such a figure. Many individuals are in perfectly good health, with no constipation, with an intake of only 10 g dietary fibre.

To achieve the increase, the dietary guidelines suggest higher intakes of fruit, vegetables, and whole grain cereals. The types of dietary fibre differ between these sources, and have different physiological effects, so a mixture of sources in desirable. If the guidelines are followed for reducing fat and sugar, the energy content of the diet will have to be made up with other foods to satisfy an individual's requirements. It is suggested in the guidelines that these are replaced with starchy foods such as bread (particularly whole grain, which is rich in dietary fibre) and potatoes.

Salt

Since the publication of the COMA Report in 1984, the evidence linking a high salt intake to the incidence of CHD has become weaker. The hypothesis was based on data from certain genetic strains of rats, which, if fed a high-salt diet from birth, develop hypertension (high blood pressure) later in life. Based on this model, it was suggested that some people (estimated at about 15% of the population) were genetically inclined to develop high blood pressure after years on a high-salt diet. There is no doubt that, in the UK, we have an unnecessarily high intake of salt, as, physiologically, human beings need one gram of sodium chloride per day and in practice we ingest 10–12 grams. However, attempts by medical practitioners to improve the blood pressure of their hypertensive patients by reducing their intake of salt have often proved unsuccessful. These results have cast doubt on the role of salt in the development of hypertension, although in fact, they do not invalidate the hypothesis.

Alcohol

There is no doubt that excessive alcohol is harmful, but there is some discussion on the benefit of moderate amounts. A plot of clinical findings against alcohol intake results in a J-shaped curve (Fig. 1.5), i.e. a small intake is beneficial compared with none, but as intake increases, so do the harmful consequences.

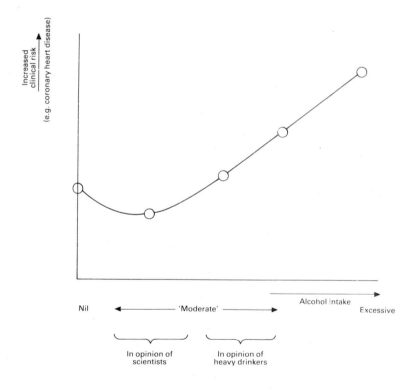

Fig. 1.5 — Relationship between intake of alcohol and clinical risk.

However, more recently, it has been suggested that the 'zero group' in Figure 1.5 includes people who cannot tolerate alcohol or who have had to stop consuming it for medical reasons and, therefore, the higher incidence of clinical effects compared with those with moderate intakes is misleading.

Impact of dietary guidelines on eating habits

So, it is clear from the above discussion that there is scope for a continuing debate about the validity of the dietary guidelines. However, since these dietary changes cannot do any harm and may well do some good, most nutritionists consider that there is every reason so to advise the public.

How much of this is getting over? Are people really changing their habits? The way this is viewed depends on whether one is an optimist or a pessimist. The optimist looks at a glass of beer and says it is half full, while a pessimist says it is half empty. So, if you consider that people are not changing their habits fast enough then you are a pessimist; but on the other hand, the optimist will see that quite a lot of changes have taken place in the few years since the publication of the 1984 COMA Report. Although there have been many radio and television programmes and the publication of much advertising and information material, local Area Health Authorities have only recently begun their campaigns.

Changes in consumption patterns of individual food items

With the manufacture of more palatable forms of wholemeal bread, its consumption has increased considerably at the expense of white. Despite the paucity of the evidence on the benefits to health of lowering the salt content, food manufacturers have been making efforts to reduce the salt in some of their products. In particular, bakers are gradually reducing the salt content of bread, so that people have time to become accustomed to any change in taste. In fact, desire for high levels of salt in the diet appears to be a matter of habit. This is shown in the following example. An experiment in Oslo commenced with a group of people taking 10 g of salt per day. They were transferred to a diet with only 2 g of salt per day for two weeks and then allowed to return to their normal diet. The diet they subsequently selected supplied 6 g of salt per day. Therefore, after only two weeks of training of the palate they wanted much less salt.

It is quite possible to alter people's likes and dislikes if only they are prepared to try a new product. It has certainly happened with milk. One fifth of all the milk consumed in the UK in 1989 was skimmed or semi-skimmed, in place of whole milk. Purchases of sugar have been falling steadily over several years, but at the same time, more foods containing sugar are being purchased, so that overall there is only a small reduction, about 1% per year, in sugar consumption. Sales of bread spread, so-called yellow fats, show an increase in the consumption of margarine at the expense of butter (Table 1.4). This is presumably influenced by price as well as for health reasons.

Changes in eating patterns

The general advice to reduce the consumption of fats has had little overall effect. The average total fat intake fell by about 6% between 1980 and 1986, but since this was accompanied by a reduction in total food intake, there was no change in the percentage of energy derived from fats (Table 1.4). There has, however, been an increase in the polyunsaturate:saturate ratio (P/S ratio) due to an increased proportion of vegetable oils.

The Health and Lifestyle Survey of 1987 (Whichelow, 1989) reported that of 9000 persons interviewed, more were still using butter and only a relatively small proportion

Table 1.4 — Changes in fat consumption in the UK recorded in the National Food
Survey

	1975	1980	1986
Total fat (g/head/day)		106	99
Butter (g/head/day)	22.9		9.3
Margarine (g/head/day)	10.7		17.1
% of dietary energy		42.3	42.5
P/S ratio		0.24	0.35

P/S, polyunsaturated fatty acids:saturated fatty acids.

were using margarines rich in polyunsaturates (PUFA). At that time, the special low-fat
spreads (40% fat compared with butter) and margarines (at 80% fat), and the more recent
25% fat products, had only a very small share of the market (Table 1.5).

Table 1.5 — 1989 Health and Lifestyle Survey in the UK: percentage of respondents
using various fat spreads ($n = 9003$)

	Men	Women
Butter	40	41
Margarine	33	28
High-PUFA margarine	16	15
Low-fat margarine	4	11

PUFA, polyunsaturates.
Source: Whichelow (1989)

What is more surprising is that only a minority of men with a family history of CHD
were using the low-fat and the PUFA spreads. Table 1.6 shows (in brackets), the
corresponding figures for men with a family history of CHD. The only statistically
significant difference in high PUFA spread intake was between those who had a family
history of CHD ('yes' in Table 1.6) and those without such a history, was for manual
workers.

Table 1.6 — 1987 Health and Lifestyle Survey in UK: Percentage use of low fat and
high-PUFA spreads by men with and without a personal or family history of coronary
heart disease (family history is in brackets)

	With History of CHD	High-PUFA	Low-fat	None
Non-manual	Yes	28 (24)	14 (10)	4 (5)
	No	20 (20)	10 (10)	4 (3)
Manual	Yes	18 (16)	7 (7)	4 (2)
	No	12 (12)	7 (7)	3 (3)

PUFA, polyunsaturates.
Source: Whichelow (1989)

CONCLUSION

The 'eating for health' campaign in the United Kingdom has been in progress for only about five years. No one problem can ever have been given so much publicity. At a guess, there must have been about 400 television and radio programmes on this topic over these past five years, many of them specifically aimed at diet and heart disease. In addition, there have been published on the subject hundreds of articles in magazines and several popular books, together with leaflets from many retailers. Despite this high profile for the campaign, dietary change in the UK has been very slow.

It is clear that people respond much better to close supervision with individual advice. In one controlled survey by the magazine *Which* and recently reported in the *Journal of Human Nutrition and Dietetics* (Bradley and Theobald, 1988), individual advice on diet was given to 28 individuals. The subjects reduced fat, sugar and salt in their diets, but, even then, did not increase the dietary fibre content. It seems that increasing the dietary fibre is more difficult to accomplish than the other changes recommended.

There are many other reports which show, not surprisingly, the greater effectiveness of individual and repeated advice compared with general exhortation. It should always be remembered that cost has a very big impact on consumer food choice and therefore on diet, which, in turn, influences health. The question is, 'Are economics more important in maintaining health than all our knowledge of nutrition and food science put together?'

REFERENCES

Benton, D. and Roberts, G. (1988) Effect of vitamin and mineral supplementation on intelligence of a sample of school children. *Lancet* **i**, 140–143.

Bradley, A. and Theobald, A. (1988) The effect of dietary modification as defined by NACNE on the eating habits of 28 people, *Journal of Human Nutrition and Dietetics.* **1**, 105–114.

DHSS (Department of Health and Social Security) (1979) *Recommended daily amounts of food energy and nutrients for groups of people in the United Kingdom.* Report on Health and Social Subjects No. 15. HMSO, London.

DHSS (1984) *Diet and cardiovascular disease.* The 'COMA Report'. *Report on Health and Social Subjects No. 28.* HMSO, London

Hopkins, P. N. and Williams, R. R. (1981) A survey of 246 suggested coronary risk factors. *Atherosclerosis* **40**, 1–52.

McGovern, D. (1977) *Dietary goals for the United States*, Select Committee on Nutrition and Human Needs, Government Printing Office, Washington, D.C.

NACNE (National Advisory Committee on Nutrition Education) (1983) *Proposals for nutritional guidelines for health education in Britain*: Discussion paper. Health Education Council, London.

Naismith, D. J., Nelson, M., Burley, V. L. and Gatenby S. J. (1988) Can children's intelligence be increasee by vitamin and mineral supplements? *Lancet* **ii**, 335.

Passmore R. and Eastwood M.A. (1986) *Davidson and Passmore: Human Nutrition and Dietetics.* 8th edition. Churchill Livingstone, Edinburgh.

Whichelow, M. J. (1989) Choice of spread by a random sample of the British population. *European Journal of Clinical Nutrition.* **43**, 1–10.

2

Assessment of the nutriture of the population

Hugh Sinclair

INTRODUCTION: THE DEVELOPMENT OF NUTRITIONAL SCIENCE
Although food science and nutrition are regarded these days as young disciplines, interest in these subjects preceded the scientific study of medicine and biochemistry. Medicine arose from noticing what patients ate, and whether particular foods madethem feel better or worse. However, as science only progresses as rapidly as the means to measure change, there was little proper investigation of food and nutritional science until developments in chemistry had taken place.

Chemistry, as distinct from alchemy, started with Robert Boyle (1627–1692) in the middle of the 17th century, and advanced with the discovery of gases. Carbon dioxide was discovered by the Scottish chemist Black (1728–1799) in 1754 when he was only 26 years old; Joseph Priestley (1733–1804) discovered oxygen in 1774; and then there were the contributions at the end of the 18th century — particularly from Lavoisier (1743–1794), whom most people would regard as being the greatest biochemist there has ever been.

Towards the end of the 1700s was a glorious period in the development of science. There were three scientists, Lavoisier, Priestley and Spallanzani (1729–1799), who were from very different backgrounds, who greatly influenced scientific thought and who met to exchange ideas. Lavoisier was a French aristocrat who was beheaded in the French Revolution in 1794. Priestley was a Unitarian minister in Birmingham, who supported the French Revolution; because of this support, a mob burnt his house down and he had to flee to America. Spallanzani was the Abbé of Pavia in Italy and the first person to show that biochemical processes proceeded optimally at body temperature. During the long, Roman Catholic Masses he used to incubate his test tubes in his armpits. He was the first person who put human digestion — so important in nutrition — on an experimental basis. He used to swallow linen bags containing foods or sponges on the end of strings and get the monks to pull them up to recover gastric juice, which he would successfully incubate in his armpits with food. The friendship of these three totally distinct people was unique, considering their backgrounds were so different. Unfortunately this kind of communication in science is all too often lacking in our enlightened modern times.

It was only after Lavoisier had been beheaded that his discoveries were used to the fullest to sow the seeds of the subject of organic chemistry. The man that particularly progressed Lavoisier's methods was Liebig (1803–1873), one of the greatest chemists that there has ever been. Liebig by 1840 was putting organic chemistry on the map and already relating it to nutrition.

The rapidity of the development in organic chemistry and its impact on the understanding of nutrient intake is well exemplified by some work of John Dalton, whose major claim to fame is the discovery of the atom. He had a long-standing interest in diet and health. In 1831 he published a small pamphlet entitled *A series of experiments on the quantity of food eaten by a person in health, compared with the quantity of the different secretions during the same period, with chemical remarks on the several articles*. Two pages of this pamphlet, including the first page, can be seen in Plates 2.1(a) and 2.1(b).

Dalton states in this publication that forty years earlier in his career he had wanted to study medicine, but he had no money to do so. Nevertheless, he retained an interest in matters to do with the body and proceeded to experiment on himself. He weighed daily everything he ate at different times of the year and collected his excreta and weighed them. In 1790 there was little he could do with such data, as there was no organic chemistry and the components of food were not known. So he put all those results away in a drawer, and in 1830, when organic chemistry had suddenly blossomed, he took out his data and was able to translate them into carbon, hydrogen, nitrogen and oxygen.

Thus, with the developments in organic chemistry, nutritional science moved along very quickly. By the turn of this century it was well advanced. The year 1863 had seen the publication of a most remarkable report — the first real scientific study of diets. In the United Kingdom there was a cotton famine and people were dying because they had no money, not because there was no food. As a consequence, the Ministry of Health did something that had never been done in any country in the world up to that point. It decided to investigate the matter scientifically. The cooperation of Edward Smith, a doctor in London, was sought to undertake a study to determine:

(1) What is the least cost per head per week for which food can be bought in such quantity and such quality as will avert starvation diseases of the unemployed population?

(2) What, with special reference to health, would be the most useful expenditure for a weekly minimum allowance granted exclusively for the purchase of food?

(3) What, if the government would provide a little more money, would be the most useful expenditure on food?

Therefore, the aim of the study was to determine how much money the average person must have weekly to avoid starvation and if the government made available that minimum amount weekly, on what foods it should be spent to achieve a survival diet.

(a)

A SERIES OF EXPERIMENTS

ON THE

QUANTITY OF FOOD,

Taken by a Person in Health,

COMPARED WITH THE QUANTITY OF THE DIFFERENT
SECRETIONS DURING THE SAME PERIOD;

WITH

CHEMICAL REMARKS ON THE SEVERAL ARTICLES.

BY JOHN DALTON, F. R. S.

Read March 5th, 1830.

DURING my residence at Kendal, nearly 40 years ago, I had at one time an inclination to the study of medicine, with a view to future practice in the medical profession. It was on this account chiefly, but partly from my own personal interest in knowing the causes of disease and of health, that I was prompted to make such investigations into the animal economy as my circumstances and situation at the time would allow. I had met with some account of Sanctorius' weighing chair and of his finding the quantity of insensible perspiration compared with

(b)

An aggregate of the articles of food consumed in the fourteen days is given below; and the mean proportions for one day are also given, neglecting small fractions.

	Consumption in 14 Days.		Consumption in 1 Day.
Bread, ...	163 *oz. avoird.*	....	12 *oz. avoird.*
Oat-cake, ...	79	....	6
Oat-meal, ...	12	....	1
Butcher's Meat,	54½	....	4
Potatoes, ...	130	....	9
Pastry, ...	55	....	4
Cheese, ...	32	.... ·	2
Total,	525½ Solids		38 Solids

2 Q

Plate 2.1 — Extracts from John Dalton's pamphlet published in 1831, showing his keen interest in matters nutritional. (a) The first page of the pamphlet. (b) An entry of food he consumed over a 14-day period

Edward Smith's superb study states that an allowance of 2 shillings a person weekly was necessary [about £0.10 in 1989]. The effects of inflation are apparent in a recent National Food Survey report (MAFF, 1987) which shows that the average amount spent in the UK is now over £10 a person weekly.

It is a sad fact that most nutritional advances have have been made because governments have given impetus to research in the face of war and, as soon as the war is over, nutrition is forgotten. In 1903 there was a report of a Royal Commission on physical training in Scotland. It was realized that men called up for the Boer War were in a poor physical state and a commission was set up to investigate the problem. The work culminated in a Parliamentary report of 'an Interdepartmental Committee on Physical Deterioration' (1904). It stated that large numbers of men called up for the armed forces were rejected on medical grounds. It was a natural progression that concern about nutrition of young men should lead to concern about the nutrition of children. Shortly after this report was published, school meals (1906) and the medical inspection of children (1907) were introduced.

ASSESSMENT OF NUTRITURE

The nutriture (state of nutrition) of à person is not the same as the physical state, as defects from past malnutriture (e.g. rachitic deformities) are irrelevant. Nutritional and non-nutritional factors influencing various states of health are shown in Fig. 2.1.

In the assessment of the nutriture of an individual, we have to be careful that we are assessing the current state of a person's nutrition and not past defects, such as rachitic deformities. There are various degrees of nutriture, ranging from one extreme to the other: excess, normal, poor, latent malnutriture, clinical malnutriture and death. However, apart from overt malnutriture and death, there is great difficulty in deciding what we mean when saying that a person is in a normal state of nutrition. The four customary definitions of normality of nutriture are:

(1)   *Perfection*. A person is normal if he or she is perfect — i.e. there is no defect. This might be interpreted to mean that a person who was perfect would stand the best possible chance of good health. However, sometimes slight defects happen to be an advantage; for example, if a person is deficient in thiamin then he or she is more resistant to polio.

(2)   *Absence of active disease or pathology*. If this is the criterion for normality then how are dental caries and acne vulgaris classified? In the case of dental caries, most people in the UK could be said to have the disease, although it is much less common in Third World countries.

        During the Second World War, the author, whilst engaged in work with the Canadian Air Force, had the opportunity of living with and studying the health and diet of Eskimos. At the time, there was no dental caries among the Eskimos, although their teeth were ground down because they chewed bones. The women chewed skins to make them more malleable for making canoes and shoes. Unfortunately, since the early 1950s, Americans have colonized Eskimos, and introduced alcohol, sugar, cigarettes and, of course, the contraceptive pill. Now,

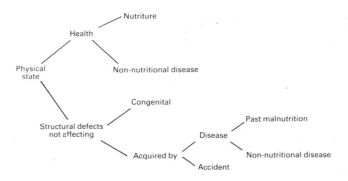

Fig. 2.1 — Nutritional and non-nutritional influences on health.

dental caries is rampant in children — higher than in the UK. (Incidentally, whereas no cancer has been recorded in an Eskimo until 1952 when a single case was found, now cancer of the cervix is extremely common, as well as other forms of cancer.)

(3)   *Statistical distribution.* The range of the physiological requirements of a given nutrient for a population group subsample, between plus and minus the standard deviation of the mean, includes 68% of the population. If this range is is extended to two standard deviations, the range includes 95% of the population (see Chapter 1). This concept is used in defining most Recommended Daily Amounts (RDA), and is based on the customary medical statistical concept that in any biochemical measurement on an individual (for example, the protein content of blood plasma), any particular parameter is only regarded as normal if it is within plus or minus twice the standard deviation of the mean for a given population.

There are difficulties with this concept however, if the mean value for the population is high. A good example is cholesterol. In most reports the view is taken that a plasma cholesterol level of over 200 mg/dl (5.3 mmol/l) is undesirable. However, the average level for adults in the UK is much above this (see Chapter 7). Thus it may not be an easy matter to fix a scale of normality merely by what is found in the population.

(4)   *Physiological function.* A person may be regarded as normal if the level of nutriture allows him or her to perform their usual functions in their usual environment.

How do we decide if a person is getting enough food?
Inadequate ingestion or absorption of food, leads to:

(a) diminished bodily reserves, which in turn, leads to:
(b) impaired function of the body, which leads to:
(c) anatomical lesions.

Whereas inadequate ingestion may be studied by economic or dietary methods, (a) can be investigated by biochemical methods, (b) by physiological methods and (c) by clinical examination.

Calculating *minimum cost diets* (i.e. how much money you must have in order to buy a proper diet) is a waste of ime. I had to assess the nutritional state of the population for the Ministry of Health during the 1939—1945 war, and in my university of Oxford, there was a lady who spent the entire war sitting at a desk calculating minimum cost diets. If I remember rightly, she concluded that it was about 12 shillings per person per week. It did not contribute to the war effort at all, although this kind of exercise does keep economists busy.

The best way to assess whether people are getting sufficient food is to consider how malnutrition arises. Perhaps a person may not have sufficient food, although in the UK any undernutrition is usually due to ignorance rather than a lack of money to spend on food. Alternatively, a person who is malnourished may not be eating the right diet; it may be unbalanced or deficient in one or more nutrient. These latter possibilities should be able to be detected by a study of dietary intake in comparison with a standard for dietary intake — normally in the form of Recommended Daily Amounts or Allowances (RDA).

If people are eating a wrong diet, then the composition of the body is going to change. For example, if they are eating too little ascorbic acid, then the level of ascorbic acid in the body will fall and this will be reflected in the blood level, which can be determined by chemical analysis.

Following biochemical changes, and perhaps quite a long time after, there will be anatomical changes and clinical lesions — e.g. sore tongue, rough dry skin — and one should be able to detect these by clinical examination. Along with the clinical examination, it is usual to include somatometric (anthropometric) measurements such as height and weight and other measurements of bodily dimensions.

Methods of dietary investigation
One can investigate diets in three different ways:

(a)   *On a population basis.* In this method the food imported into a country is recorded and any food exports are subtracted, then food produced in the country is added and the total food available is divided by the total number in the civilian population to obtain a *per capita* figure for food intake. Clearly the method is extremely rough-and-ready. Although the Food and Agriculture Organization of the United Nations [FAO] does, in fact, publish figures for the average *per capita* consumption in different populations on a yearly basis, this approach is very crude because of the lack of precision in data collection.

The limitations of such a method are illustrated by problems encountered with it during the 1939–1945 war. An Allied commission was set up to produce what were called 'food consumption levels' for the civilian population of the UK, USA and Canada, and I was made a member. To aid this commission, a group of civil servants spent a considerable time trying to decide if the merchant navy were civilian population or not. I pointed out that it was pointless being so pedantic as there were five million dogs in the country whose food consumption had been completely overlooked!

(b)   *On an institutional or family basis.* Although this approach can be used in an institution such as a school or hospital, it is more familiar in the UK applied on a family basis as the National Food Survey (NFS: MAFF, 1952 onwards). The NFS report has been published each year since 1952 and data are gathered by the 'inventory and purchase' method. It is necessary to record food stored in the house at the start of the week, all the food purchased during the week and how much is paid for it. The number of people eating meals during the week is also recorded and whether any occupant has taken a packed lunch to eat outside the home. Home-grown food is recorded and at the end of the week food stored in the home is again recorded.

In this way, an estimate of the food consumed by that household during the week can be made. Weighing indices are then used to calculate food consumed by different members of the household (young children obviously eating less). Waste is not normally recorded, and neither is food fed to pets, so the method is by no means perfect. Nevertheless, it is useful for assessing eating trends over time. As both consumption and expenditure are recorded, there are many uses for the NFS, including commercial ones. However, one of the major drawbacks of the NFS is that it only concerns food consumed in the home and ignores food consumed outside the home.

(c)   *By individual weighed dietary survey.* In this method the individual is provided with weighing scales. Before a meal a plate is placed on the scales, which are adjusted to zero. Foods to be eaten are placed on the plate in the ready-to-eat state and their weights recorded. At the end of the meal the plate is placed back on the scales, with the inedible portions such as the plum stones, and the weights recorded. The method is very tedious, but gives a reasonably accurate estimate of what an individual has eaten at a particular meal. Inaccuracies in the method arise from the individuals becoming too conscious of their intake and perhaps eating less than normal in consequence.

Translation of food into nutrients

Having obtained weights of individual foods eaten, it is necessary to translate these into nutrients. This is usually done using composition of foods tables, such as the very useful ones of *McCance and Widdowson* (Paul and Southgate, 1978). It is important when using such tables to understand clearly at what stage in food preparation the food was weighed. In the NFS, the weight of the food is the weight 'as purchased' (AP). In the case of potatoes this would be with earth and skin. Food 'as purchased' is very different from what people actually eat. Fig. 2.2 serves to illustrate this point.

If the weight of the food eaten is recorded AP (Fig. 2.2), the food provider in the household is going to take off two things from that, which are called inedible waste. The first is preparation waste — perhaps the skins of the potatoes and certainly the earth. Then secondly, there is the waste on the plate — the stones of fruit, the inedible gristle of the meat and the bones of chicken, etc. These items have been weighed but are not going to be eaten. So their weight must be subtracted from the AP weight. What we are really interested in is to estimate the amount of food which is actually absorbed into the body. In addition to the losses already mentioned, there are going to be losses in cooking —

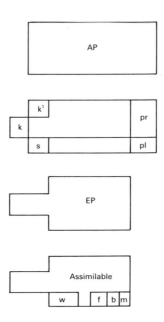

$$E = P\text{-}(pr + pl) - (k^1 + s) + k$$
$$N = E - (f + m + b) - u$$

Where:-
$P =$ food as purchased (AP, e.g. potatoes with skin and earth);
$pr + pl =$ inedible waste, preparation and plate (e.g. earth and plum stones);
$k^1 + s =$ edible waste (losses in cooking and serving);
$k =$ additions in cooking, E = food as eaten (EP)
$N =$ assimilable nutrients;
$f =$ indigestible; m = metabolic products (bile acids, gut cells)
$b =$ microflora; u = losses in urine (e.g. urea).

Digestibility $= E - (f + b)$, availability $= E - (f + b + m)$.

Fig. 2.2 — Differences between food as purchased (AP), food as eaten (edible portion, EP), digestibility, availability and assimilabilty.

some may be left in the saucepan or other cooking vessel. There may also be loss in serving — some will be left on the dishes. Other ingredients may be added in food preparation which have not been recorded in food AP.

Food digestibility, absorption and Atwater factors

Even if due allowance is made for all the points mentioned in the previous paragraph we still may not have arrived at the figure for the amount of food absorbed and utilized by the body. To calculate energy intake, account must be taken of indigestible food which is lost in the faeces and food which is not completely utilized by the body (protein, which is only oxidized by the body as far as urea, not the complete oxidation to nitrous gases which would happen if it were burnt in air).

These latter points were described by the greatest American nutritionist — Atwater (1844–1907). He realized that not only were some substances in the food indigestible, but that these were supplemented in the gut by the excretion of endogenous products of metabolism. Thus endogenous cholesterol and bile salts, which appear in the gut, and mucosal cells of the gut are constantly being shed and excreted.

Several textbooks quote energy conversion figures produced by the a great German nutritionist Rubner (1854–1932), which were 4.1 for carbohydrate, 4.1 for protein and 9.3 for fat. These figures were worked out on a man, a boy, a baby and a dog. An allowance was made for losses of nitrogen from protein in urine and faeces, but not for losses in faeces from fat or carbohydrate. This work in no way matched that of Atwater: indeed, dogs metabolize protein better than man. Therefore, Rubner's figures were not very accurate.

Atwater's general conversion figures for carbohydrates, protein and fat were 4.0, 4.0 and 8.9 (which he interpreted to be as near as 9.0 as makes no difference). Because these figures are whole numbers, many textbooks have assumed that Atwater produced rough figures, but this was by no means the case. The *Atwater factors* as they are now known, were produced around the turn of this century on three adult American men, with the greatest of care. Atwater fed his volunteers on single food items, for example, nothing but potatoes, then nothing but cabbage, then nothing but beef. During these trials, he collected urine and faeces and went to great lengths to obtain precise data. The experiments of Atwater are regarded these days as some of the most meticulous and detailed ever done in the history of nutrition. Atwater factors are still in use today, though strictly, they are only general factors applicable to American diets at the end of the last century.

Comparison of nutrient intake with requirements or allowances

A classical assessment of daily energy requirements was made in the UK during the 1939–1945 war. Britain was losing the war at the time, because the incompetent Minister of Food refused to introduce food rationing. Uninvited, the Royal Society set up a committee, which included Gowland Hopkins (Nobel Prize for vitamin research) and other distinguished people. They published, in 1946, a report: *The Food Supplies of the United Kingdom — a Report of a Committee of the Royal Society*.

In this report the daily diet of an average male (soldier doing light work in barracks used as example) was specified as required to contain 100 g protein, 100 g fat and 500 g carbohydrate in the food as purchased. This would give 3390 kilocalories daily, since they used Rubner's factors, and they stated that no account of losses of digestion had been made. Since their foods were AP about 10% should be deducted to give foods EP. (In fact, the committee were confused about the application of Rubner factors — as the Rubner factors incorporate allowance for digestibility of protein.)

So they were allowing a soldier an energy intake of around 3000 available kilocalories, which is regarded as unnecessarily high these days. Their value for protein would also now be regarded as too high — most recommendations are now around 1 g per kg body weight, which gives a figure of about 65 g daily for a man. There is no need to modify protein intake according to the energy demands of the body. I was engaged in feeding Germans after the 1939–1945 war in Germany, and the miners were all demanding extra protein rations. In fact there was no justification for this, as muscular work is not carried out at the expense of body protein.

In addition, we would now regard 100 g fat as being too high and not compatible with good health. There are several influential reports which have strongly recommended reducing fat intake to reduce the risk of CHD, especially saturated fat intake (see Chapters 1 and 7).

RDA — Recommended Daily Amounts (Recommended Dietary Allowances) of nutrients

In the USA RDA stands for *Recommended Dietary Allowances*, and in the UK for *Recommended Daily Amounts*. One use of RDAs is as a yardstick for comparison against nutrient intake of a particular human group. As mentioned above, the intake of individuals can be assessed by weighing foods eaten and then translating these into nutrients using a composition of foods tables.

To use RDAs sensibly it is important to realize how they are devised. RDAs are usually based on the statistical concept of normality — i.e. the normal distribution of any particular parameter which you might care to measure in a healthy population (see also discussion in Chapter 1). In statistical terms, the normal distribution can be represented by the Gaussian (or normal) distribution curve. Although the use of the normal distribution is common, problems can arise in its use.

With such measurements as human height the use of the normal distribution is straightforward. Let us take a group of adult women whose average height may be 5ft 6in. Obviously, there are a number of people shorter and taller than the mean. Plus or minus twice the standard deviation of the mean value should give us the range of most (about 95%) of the group.

The problem comes in the use of the normal distribution in attempting to recommend energy intake of groups. For any group we are now in a quandary, as some requirements of the population group will be higher and some lower than the mean requirement — so how are recommended daily allowances set? The problem of fixing RDAs for energy is that people should not be encouraged to eat more than their requirements, as obesity may result, which is a hazard to health. With nutrients apart from energy it is common for any particular group to set the RDA at the requirements of the mean of the group plus two standard deviations, because with nutrients apart from energy a little excess is of no consequence, therefore it is better to err on the safe side. For energy, as obesity is a risk to health, for any particular human group the RDA is set at the mean value for the requirement of the group.

The first edition of the USA RDA tables was published in 1943. There have been new editions since then at the approximate rate of two per decade, with the ninth edition published in 1980. There has been no edition since 1980, because nutritionists and policy makers are squabbling about new recommendations, mainly over vitamin A and whether a higher level of it should be introduced into the RDA to act as a preventative against cancer.

It is important to realize that RDAs are not figures written on tablets of stone. In fact, they are extremely rough and ready. I happened to be a British Observer in the USA when the first RDAs were drawn up, and the figure for ascorbic acid was finally accepted as 75 mg per adult person per day. That figure was derived in this way: a distinguished person (Professor McHenry) would not accept any figure above 50 mg, and another distinguished person (Dr Glen King) would not accept any figure below 100 mg, so the committee agreed on the figure of 75 mg, which is regarded by naive people as a sacrosanct figure. That process of deriving RDAs is not nutritional science, but guesswork!

Similarly, in setting the UK RDA for vitamin C for adults some figure had to be published. It was known that 6 mg of ascorbic acid daily will cure scurvy, but in the UK it was thought that most diets should have about 20 mg, so a bit more was added on and 30 mg was accepted. There is clearly room for improvement in the rationale for setting RDAs! The last UK RDAs were produced in 1979, and they are now being revised.

Biochemical measurement of nutriture
Nutriture (nutritional status) can be determined biochemically either for people on their normal diets or after test doses of certain nutrients. Nutriture is often measured by carrying out chemical analyses of tissues or body fluids for nutrients or body fluid components affected by nutrients: such as albumin, haemoglobin, ascorbic acid. Alternatively, products of metabolism may be measured (such as the level of pyruvate, etc.) or enzymes (such as transketolase for thiamin). Tissues or fluids examined can be:

(a) Blood erythrocytes (red cells) or leucocytes (white cells), muscle, adipose tissue, hair, nails, buccal cells. These tissues may show the longer-term effects of nutrient intake.

(b) Blood plasma or serum.

(c) Urine or other fluids (e.g. cerebro-spinal fluid, sweat).

It is the usual procedure to examine blood or blood components, but often information from these samples is taken to represent the entire body, which it may not necessarily do.

(Some nutritionists have commented that although it is all right to take blood samples from adults, as their permission can be obtained, it is unethical to take blood from children. I have been taking blood samples from children in different countries of the world for years. Not to be allowed to take blood samples from children would impose an intolerable restraint on nutritionists seeking to help those children. In fact, normally a child does not know when one is taking a drop of blood; it does not even hurt, as the usual practice for children is to prick the ear lobe. In my opinion, it is totally ethical and in the child's interest to know that its nutriture is adequate.)

There are micromethods for analysing blood samples these days, so only very small blood samples need be taken. Apart from taking a little blood for haemoglobin analyses, a drop of blood is drawn into a capillary tube, which is sealed at both ends by flame, or with wax. The tube is then spun in a centrifuge so that the red cells will sediment, with the white cells in the middle and plasma at the top. All three of these blood constituents can be used to determine nutriture, but individually may give a different picture of changes.

For example, on a diet deficient in ascorbic acid, the amount of ascorbic acid in the blood plasma will decline rapidly. The amount of ascorbic acid in plasma in a normal state of nutrition will be about 0.5 mg/dl. That immediately drops to zero in about 2–3 weeks, and the urinary level also drops to zero very rapidly. But the ascorbic acid content of living cells of the body such as white cells is high and falls only slowly, even with a diet deficient in ascorbic acid — until about 120 days after the commencement of the low ascorbic acid diet, when it falls to about zero and the first clinical signs of scurvy appear. Therefore, ascorbic acid in urine and blood plasma can indicate only recent past intake, but low level in leucocytes can give more information over a longer term. A low level in these cells, therefore, would be very detrimental for health.

For some measurements, such as trace elements, samples of hair or nail can be used. Also biopsies can be valuable. I carried out adipose tissue biopsies during the experiment in which I ate only an Eskimo diet of fish and seal. Adipose tissue biopsy is very simple to make and can yield some very useful information. A wide-bore needle is inserted into the tissue and a little saline is injected, the needle is moved around a bit and some fat sucked out. These samples can be used to measure the fatty acid profile, which, as adipose tissue only turns over slowly, would reflect the fatty acid profile of the diet in the preceding few months. The turnover actually depends on the amounts of body fat stored, as obese people will get alteration in adipose tissue only very slowly. On an Eskimo diet, there is almost no dietary linoleic acid, as this fatty acid is almost absent in fish and seal meat. This led in me to a dramatic loss of this fatty acid in adipose tissue, which level rose after return to a normal diet (see Fig. 5.8 in Chapter 5).

Although changes in adipose tissue fatty acid profiles are usually very slow, changes within the blood are much more rapid, indicating the dietary fat profile of the last few days only. Most fatty acids are transported in the blood from the liver to peripheral tissues as triacylglycerols in VLDL (very low density lipoprotein) and LDL (low density lipoprotein). (These terms are explained in Chapter 7.) On the other hand, the fatty acid profiles of red blood cells more closely reflect the dietary intake of the last 2 or 3 months of diet.

Functional changes as tests of nutriture
Functional tests include visual acuity, dark adaptation, capillary fragility, ergometry and dynamometry. With the exception of dark adaptation, these tests have limited application for the measurement of body nutrient status; indeed, the so-called endurance tests are useless.

The misapplication of one of these tests can be judged by the following example. In the 1939–1945 war, the Ministry of Health introduced the 'Bar Test' for school children.

A broom handle or equivalent was fixed horizontally to supports and children were required to hang from it and the time that they hung was measured. This time was alleged to be proportional to nutritional status. However, it was obvious that if there was a competitive element the children hung on for much longer. The Bar Test was in use at the end of the war. I observed, during the relief of the Dutch famine, that starving children did not hang on the bar for very long because they knew that when they dropped off, the series of examinations was over and they would be given chocolate — something they had heard about, but not experienced.

There is only one useful functional test and this is the ability to see in the dark (dark adaptation). This ability is lost in severe vitamin A deficiency, as this vitamin is required for the formation of rhodopsin, the visual pigment of rods, the retinal cells operating at low light intensity. Dark adaptation can be measured with a dark adaptometer (see Plate 2.2), which is an apparatus with a camera shutter in front of a torch bulb. Behind the shutter is a neutral wedge, which is opaque at one end and transparent at the other. The wedge is capable of dimming the light to a varying extent, depending on its position. A small red light shines at 6° above the aperture of the shutter. First the patient has to adapt, by sitting in the dark for 30 minutes. The patient is then asked to gaze at the red light and asked when he/she can see a flash of light below this as the shutter is opened. The dark adaptation can be measured by the position of the wedge. (The red light is used because it does not affect the ability of the rods to function in the dark and ensures that the same area of the retina is being tested. Incidentally, while a person is sitting in the dark for 30 minutes, a diet history and a blood sample can be taken using red light, as no one faints on seeing blood the same colour as everything else!)

Anatomical (including somatometric) nutriture tests
Under this heading one may include Body Mass Index (W/h^2), skin thickness, nail growth, mortality and vital statistics as well as methods of examination including the so-called 'Glance' method.

Medical examination of school children in the UK to assess their state of health started in 1907 and was prompted by the poor state of health of recruits for the South African War, as mentioned above. In 1913 the Dumfermline Scale was used for assessing the state of nutrition of children. This was the first time in history that anyone had bothered to try to measure whether children were adequately fed. Height, weight, posture, attention, general appearance of various parts of the body, including mucous membranes were recorded.

In 1934 the Board of Education drew up a list of nine criteria for medical officers to use in schools when undertaking medical examination of children. This was nicknamed the 'Glance' method. By 1938 this method had been discredited, owing mainly to the work of R H Jones, a statistician, who found that one school medical officer would classify a child in category A (excellent nutriture) while another officer would classify the same child in category D (bad). Clearly the Glance method was not objective, but at least attention was paid to the nutrition of children.

One measurement which did appear to have some useful nutritional basis was the measurement of weight and height. This was shown to be different, in different parts of the country, in children of the same age and in adults, although the exact nutritional significance of that was not entirely understood then and is still not today.

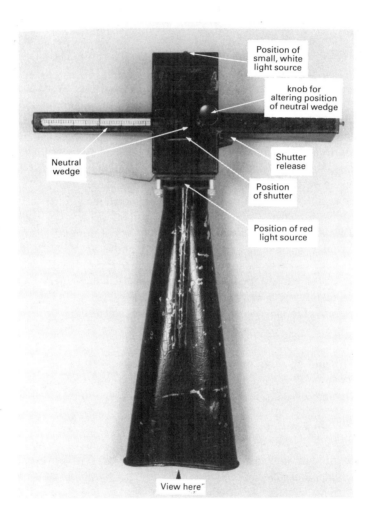

Position of
small, white
light source

knob for
altering position
of neutral wedge

Neutral
wedge

Shutter
release

Position
of shutter

Position of red
light source

View here"

Plate 2.2 — A dark adaptometer. An instrument which measures ability to see in the dark, which is related to vitamin A nutriture (the only useful functional test in nutrition).

Skin calipers

Subcutaneous tissue is nipped in the calipers (see Plate 2.3) and the thickness of the two layers of skin and the fat recorded. This method is known to correlate very well with total amount of fat in the body. A more reliable measurement of measuring body fat is to weigh people in and out of water to determine their specific gravity, but this is reserved as a reference method, as it is not so easy to carry out. (See Chapter 6.)

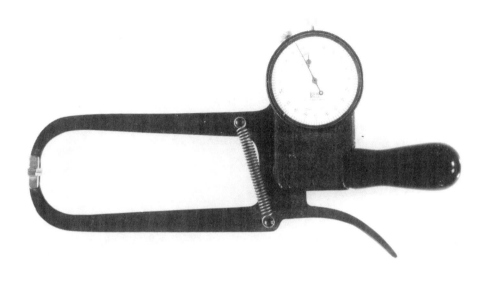

Plate 2.3 — Skin calipers: subcutaneous tissue is nipped between the arms of the calipers and the thickness of the two layers of skin is recorded on the dial.

CONCLUSION

It is very important to make sure in survey work that the data are well tabulated. Even in these days of computing, the use of the notched card system still has its merits, in that it is readily portable in the field. Each patient has a card, and various parameters during physical examination can be recorded by cutting out the appropriate holes. Later, classifying cards is easy using a knitting needle. Numbers of cards in different categories can be determined by weighing.

Before carrying out a survey it is very important to make contact with the right people, such as the head of the community and (in some cases) the witch doctor. Without their cooperation you'll get nowhere. For example, in these days we have to win the cooperation of Eskimos with cigarettes and sugar — regrettable, but necessary for success in a survey.

All the time, during such a survey, your eyes should be open to observe usual foods eaten and preparation methods, and samples should be collected for analysis whenever possible. Although it is 126 years since Edward Smith scientifically investigated the dietary relief of the Cotton Famine, only in the last half century have methods become available accurately to assess the nutriture of populations and so to attempt to alleviate starvation and malnutriture.

REFERENCES

Bigwood, E J (1939) *Guiding principles for studies on the nutrition of population.* League of Nations, Geneva.

Bingham, S. A. (1987) The dietary assessment of individuals: methods, accuracy, new techniques and recommendations. *Nutrition Abstracts and Reviews (Series A).* **57** (10), 705–742.

DHSS (1979) *Recommended daily amounts of food energy and nutrients for groups of people in the UK.* Report on Health and Social Subjects No. 15. Reprinted with revision 1981. HMSO. London.

FAO (1974) *Handbook on human nutritional requirements.* FAO Nutritional Studies No. 28. Food and Agriculture Organization of the United Nations, Rome.

FAO/WHO Joint Expert Groups:
Calcium requirements, (1961).
Requirements for vitamin A, thiamin, riboflavin and niacin (1965).
Requirements for ascorbic acid, vitamin D, vitamin B12, folate and iron (1970).
Energy and protein requirements (1973).
Food and Agricultural Organization of the United Nations, Rome.

Jelliffe, D. B. (1966) The assessment of the nutritional status of the community. WHO, Geneva.

MAFF (Ministry of Agriculture, Fisheries and Food) (1952 onwards). Household consumption and expenditure. *The National Food Survey.* HMSO, London.

Marr, J. W. (1971) Individual dietary surveys. *World Reviews of Nutrition and Dietetics.* **13**, 106–164.

Paul, A. A. and Southgate, D. A. T. (1978) *McCance and Widdowson's The composition of foods.* 4th ed. MRC Special Report Series No. 297. HMSO, London.

Sinclair, H. M. (1948) The assessment of human nutriture. *Vitamins and Hormones.* **6**, 102–162.

Sinclair, H. M. (1948) Clinical surveys and correlation with biochemical, somatometric and performance measurements. *British Journal of Nutrition.* **2**, 161–170.

Sinclair, H. M. (1964) The assessment of nutriture. In: (Witts, L. J. ed.) *Medical surveys and clinical trials..* Oxford University Press, Pp 203-219.

Truswell, A. S. (1983) Recommended Daily Intakes around the world: Part I. *Nutrition Abstracts and Reviews Series A.* **53**, 940–1015 (Part II, pp 1075–1119).

US Army, Quartermaster General (1954) *Methods for evaluation of nutritional adequacy and status.* National Academy of Science, Washington.

US Dept. HEW (1960) World Nutrition Surveys. *Public Health Report* **75**, 677–773.

US Food and Nutrition Board, NRC (1949) Nutrition surveys: their techniques and value. *Bulletin of the National Research Council,* No. 117.

US Inter-Departmental Committee on Nutrition for National Defense. (1963) *Manual for nutrition surveys.* 2nd ed. Bethesda, MD: NIH.

US National Research Council (1980) *Recommended dietary allowances.* 9th ed. Food and Nutrition Board, Academy of Sciences, NRC, Washington, DC.

3

Methods of research in human nutrition

Hugh Sinclair

Introduction

In the historical development of the science of food and nutrition, considerable contributions to knowledge were made by a number of comparatively young men. Joseph Black was 26 years old when he discovered carbon dioxide in 1754. Helmholtz was also 26 when he discovered the law of conservation of energy, which was so exceptional that it was not accepted, so he had to publish it in 1847 at his own expense. Another example was Robert Boyle, the greatest chemist there has even been, who was 29 years old when, without a University education, he settled in Oxford and was so brilliant in his experiments that all the local great men, including Christopher Wren (Professor of Mathematics), gathered around him. That was the start of what became the Royal Society. So, when you are young, and if you keep your eyes open, you can wheedle out some secret of nature, collect a Nobel Prize and spend the rest of your life drifting round the world collecting honorary degrees. It is important never to be discouraged.

OBSERVATION AND EXPERIMENT

Science is advanced in two ways: by observation and by experiment. Observation means simply watching things as they happen to occur without influencing them. Astronomy, for example, at least until recently, was purely an observational science, as mankind was not able to intervene in the stars. Until the 17th century, almost all science was observational, including food and nutritional science. About that time, experimentation was introduced and distinguished scientists then considered that mere observation was of no value. This is, of course, wrong, although there are still distinguished people today, who hold the opinion that observation serves no useful function. But there are many instances of important scientific discoveries which would not have occurred without observation. The epidemiological correlation of diet and diseases in different countries is observational and has shown that there will always be a place for observation as well as experimentation in the food and nutritional sciences.

Human food choice: observation and instruction versus instinct
In the course of evolution, human beings have used observation to determine foods which could or could not be eaten. By trial and error it was observed that certain foods were poisonous, or that certain foods were beneficial if you were ill. Information on toxic effects of plants was passed by word of mouth from one person to another, even though the precise nature of the poison was not understood. Toxicity is sometimes not recognized in foods, even by lower animals, who are often considered to be able to distinguish toxic substances by instinct. An example of this is the plant called gifblaar, which grows in parts of East Africa and Australasia. It is now known to contain fluoroacetic acid, which is an extremely toxic compound, since it blocks the tricarboxylate cycle by combining with acetyl CoA and preventing its entry into the Cycle. Animals feeding on the plant do not recognise its toxic effect, and there are many reports of the plant killing cattle that have fed on it. Indeed, the toxin is used as a rat poison.

However, not all animals are so insensitive to the hazards of toxins. It is surprising that the husky dogs of the Eskimos recognize that polar bear liver is toxic. The polar bear lives on fish and concentrates enormous quantities of vitamin A (retinol) in its liver. High doses of vitamin A are extremely toxic. We do not know how husky dogs realize that polar bear liver is toxic.

The Arctic explorer Mawson died from eating polar bear and husky dog liver when his rations ran out, showing that man does not have the foresight of the husky. The following is another example of the lack of ability of man to reject food providing inappropriately high levels of retinol. I once had a girl referred to me who had gone blind from bleeding into her eyes, had rough skin and bruises, and whose teeth and bones were breaking. I diagnosed the problem as vitamin A excess. She had come over from Ireland, where she had been told that the British winter was dreadful and that cod-liver oil was just the thing to ward off its ill effect. As she liked cod-liver oil she had been taking a bottle a day.

Rats can be very responsive to the presence of nutrients in foods. If you give two bowls of food to a thiamin-deficient rat, one bowl with a thiamin-deficient diet and the other with the addition of a trace of thiamin (so small that it could not possibly be detected by smell or taste), after just two of three trials, the rat will go straight for the one containing thiamin and use only that particular bowl. It is thought that the rat learns very quickly that one food is making it 'feel better'. At least that is the only explanation we have.

This is not an explanation that applies to calcium. It is well known that cows with milk fever (calcium deficiency caused by the high output of calcium into the milk, while the intake from grass is very low) will seek out bones and chew them — even though the animal's dentition is not well suited to chewing bones. Much better documented is the fact that lactating sows deficient in calcium will lick the whitewash off the walls of their sties. It is inconceivable that the sow will lick the wall of the sty at random and 'feel better'. Indeed, it is very difficult to understand how receiving extra calcium, even if the animal is calcium deficient, will make the animal 'feel better'. We simply do not know how these instincts operate. However, it is certain that human instinct towards foods, both negative and positive, are very poor indeed.

Great Historial Observations

The earliest observations made are written on the Kahun and Ebers papyri (1850 BC and 1600 BC), which are the earliest known medical records. In both of these it is recorded that liver is very good for night blindness. This information must have come from observation that liver in the diet would improve vision in dim light.

Observation in the nutritional sciences flourished in the school of Pythagoras (580–490 BC). Members of the school were vegetarians who made close observations on foods that made people feel ill or better. A follower of Pythagoras was Hypocrates (460–375 BC), who wrote about the merits of fibre in high-extraction flour compared with refined flour.

Galen (AD 130–200), a great medical scientist, made a special study of foods for athletes to enable them to run faster. He was medical advisor to the Roman gladiators, on whom he also carried out a number of experiments.

Vitamin C: early observations not implemented

In more recent times, observations of diet and health on long sea voyages proved invaluable in the understanding of the role of vitamin C. In fact, these observations were not only restricted to sea voyages. The Romans moving overland through Europe were thwarted in their progress into Holland, because their troups died of scurvy. It was common in the days of long sea voyages to stock up on non-perisable provisions like ship's biscuit: after some weeks there was nothing fresh to eat and scurvy broke out.

One of the best accounts of all is the voyage of Jacques Cartier to Canada in 1535. He travelled from France with three ships which became ice-bound in the St Lawrence River. Scurvy broke out: several of the crew died and all the remainder, except three or four, were severely ill. After five months one of the crew who was severely ill himself, travelled on land and returned completely well. The friendly Indians had told him that the leaves of the white cedar — pine needles — were a very good thing for this disease. We now know that these needles are a very rich source of ascorbic acid. So, 450 years ago there was a clear indication from observation that scurvy could be prevented. And yet scurvy prevailed on many subseqent voyages because the discovery was not implemented.

The classic book on scurvy is Lind's 'A treatise of the scurvy', published in 1753. It is a remarkably good book. In the preface he states that, in order to write this book, he had to 'weed out a great deal of rubbish'. He goes on to describe all the work which had been done on scurvy, including that of Jacques Cartier (Plate 3.1). He also describes his own celebrated experiment.

> 'On the 20th of May 1747, I took twelve patients in the scurvy, on board the *Salisbury* at sea. Their cases were as similar as I could have them...Two of these were ordered each a quart of cyder a-day. Two others took twenty-five drops of *elixer vitriol* [sulphuric acid] three times a-day.... Two others took two spoonfuls of vinegar three

(a)

148 *Of the prevention of the scurvy.* Part II.

preservative, and most efficacious remedy, by the experience of others.

I shall then endeavour to give it the most convenient portable form, and shew the method of preserving its virtues entire for years, so that it may be carried to the most distant parts of the world in small bulk, and at any time prepared by the sailors themselves: adding some farther directions, given chiefly with a view to inform the captains and commanders of ships and fleets, of methods proper both to preserve their own health, and that of their crew.

It will not be amiss further to observe, in what method convalescents ought to be treated, or those who are weak, and recovering from other diseases, in order to prevent their falling into the scurvy; which will include some necessary rules for resisting the beginnings of this evil, when, through want of care, or neglect, the disease is bred in a ship.

As the salutary effects of the prescribed measures will be rendered still more certain, and universally beneficial, where proper regard is had to such a state of air, diet, and regimen, as may contribute to the general intentions of preservation or cure; I shall conclude the precepts relating to the preservation of seamen, with shewing the best means of obviating many inconveniencies which attend long voyages, and of removing the several causes productive of this mischief.

The

Chap. IV. *Of the prevention of the scurvy.* 149

The following are the experiments.

On the 20th of *May* 1747, I took twelve patients in the scurvy, on board the *Salisbury* at sea. Their cases were as similar as I could have them. They all in general had putrid gums, the spots and lassitude, with weakness of their knees. They lay together in one place, being a proper apartment for the sick in the fore-hold; and had one diet common to all, viz. water-gruel sweetened with sugar in the morning; fresh mutton-broth often times for dinner; at other times light puddings, boiled biscuit with sugar, &c. and for supper, barley and raisins, rice and currants, sago and wine, or the like. Two of these were ordered each a quart of cyder a-day. Two others took twenty-five drops of *elixir vitriol.* three times a-day, upon an empty stomach; using a gargle strongly acidulated with it for their mouths. Two others took two spoonfuls of vinegar three times a-day, upon an empty stomach; having their gruels and their other food well acidulated with it, as also the gargle for their mouth. Two of the worst patients, with the tendons in the ham rigid (a symptom none of the rest had) were put under a course of sea-water. Of this they drank half a pint every day, and sometimes more or less, as it operated, by way of gentle physic. Two others had each two oranges and one lemon given them every day. These they eat with greediness, at different times, upon an empty stomach. They continued

L 3 but

(b)

176 *Of the prevention of the scurvy.* Part II.

this distemper became less frequent (g). And among the first cures recommended to the world was wine, with wormwood infused in it (h); which was afterwards long used by way of prevention in *Saxony*, where this evil was peculiarly endemic (i). Fermented vinous liquors of any kind are indeed very beneficial. But it appears by the experience of the northern *American* colonies, as also of several countries up the *Baltic* in *Europe*, &c. that genuine spruce beer is, above all others, not only an effectual preservative against it, but an excellent remedy.

The antiscorbutic virtue of the fir was, like many other of our best medicines, accidentally discovered in *Europe* (k). When the *Swedes* carried on a war against the *Muscovites*, almost all the soldiers of their army were destroyed by the true marsh or marine scurvy, having rotten gums, rigid tendons, &c. But a stop was put to the progress of this disease, by the advice of *Erbenius* the King's physician, with a simple decoction of fir-tops; by which the most deplorable cases were perfectly recovered, and the rest of the soldiers prevented from falling into it. It also proved an excellent gargle for the putrid gums. From thence this medicine came

(g) *Bruner tratt. de scorbuto.*
(h) See part 3. chap. 1. *Olaus Magnus.*
(i) See part 3. chap. 2.
(k) *Vid. Mollenbrock de arthritide vaga scorbutica*, p. 116. *Ismalleri opera*, p. 2. said by some to have occurred in the army of Uladislaus King of *Poland.*

into

Chap. IV. *Of the prevention of the scurvy.* 177

into great reputation, and the common fir, *picea major*, or *abies rubra*, was afterwards called *pinus antiscorbutica.* Pinus *sylvestris*, the mountain-pine, has likewise been found highly antiscorbutic, of which a late accident has furnished a convincing proof. In the year 1736 two squadrons of ships fitted out by the court of *Russia*, were obliged to winter in *Siberia.* One commanded by *Demetrias Laptiew*, not far from the mouth of the river *Lena*, was attacked by the scurvy. The men in their distress by chance found near them this tree growing in the mountains, and experienced it to have a most surprising antiscorbutic virtue. At the same time while *Alexius Tschirikow* was passing the winter in the river *Judoma*, where it runs into the river *Maja*, a considerable number of his men were dreadfully afflicted with that disease. After various fruitless attempts to discover a remedy able to put a stop to this cruel disaster, he at length accidentally hit also upon the pines which grew plentifully on the mountains, by which all his men were recovered in a few days. In some the medicine proved gently laxative, in others it affected the body so mildly, that its operation was scarce sensible (l).

I am inclined to believe, from the description given by *Cartier* of the *ameda* tree, with a decoction of the bark and leaves of which his crew was so speedily recovered, that it was

(l) *Gmelin flor. Sibiric.* p 181.

N the

Plate 3.1 — Extracts from Lind's classic book *A Treatise of the scurvy*, published in 1753. (a) His description of his own celebrated experiment in which he tried out a number of substances that were officially recommended at the time, including sea water, as cures for scurvy. (b) His review of previously published reports of the antiscorbutic effect of pine and fir needles, including the reports of Jacques Cartier (1535).

> times a-day. Two of the worst patients ... were put under a course
> of sea-water.... And Two others had each two oranges and one
> lemon given them every day. These they eat with greediness'.

He was trying out substances that were officially recommended at the time, including sea water, as cures for scurvy. The men treated with oranges and lemons were cured in a matter of days, while and the others were steadily getting worse. The experiment would not be accepted for publication today because there were too few subjects; but it is one of the most classic experiments ever done, although it is often misquoted.

To show how early there was knowledge of the cure for scurvy, there was a publication on the subject of scurvy even earlier than Lind's book. In the 1590s the Dutch East India Company was formed and started trading with the Far East. On the first voyage of the this Company, in 1601, many of the sailors died of scurvy, except in the ship of the Company's General, Sir James Lancaster, who had included lemons in his ship's rations and had little scurvy among his crew. This observation is recorded because in 1617 the medical officer of the Dutch East India Company, Woodall, published a book in which there is a chapter on the cure of scurvy (Plate 3.2):

> 'The use of the juice of lemons is a precious medicine and well
> tried being sound and good. Let it have chief place in the cure of
> the scurvy for it will deserve it....Some surgeons (doctors) also give
> this juice daily to men in health as a preservative which course is
> good if they have store — otherwise it is best to keep it for need.'

Thus, in 1617 there is absolutely clear evidence of how to prevent scurvy, but this knowledge was not implemented. Indeed, 150 years later, in 1744, just before Lind's book was published, Lord Anson made a voyage around the world and over half his sailors died of scurvy, which was the reason that Lind dedicated his book to Lord Anson. Sadly, it took the British Navy a further forty years before they introduced lime juice into rations as an antiscorbutic. Lime juice was used for sailors for reasons of trade. Limes were easy to come by and cheap, but lemons were not so readily available. In fact lime juice does not contain so much ascorbic acid as lemon juice.

Vitamin C instability and scurvy

It took 150 years after Lind's book was published before the mercantile marine used antiscorbutics successfully. This was not gross stupidity, but arose from the fact that the ships' surgeons were using extracted lemon or lime juice, which was found to be useless after 80 or 100 days at sea, when scurvy broke out. Without refrigeration the juice was fermenting and losing its vitamin C activity.

The Dutch attempted to tackle this problem in a most intelligent way, although it was to no avail. About 1650 they set up, in Leipzig, the first chair of organic chemistry in the world. It was agreed that the professor, Andreas Moellenbrok, should carry out research into antiscorbutics because so many sailors were dying of scurvy. He made extracts, but — this is the very important point — he had no good way of testing the efficacy of them. Extracts had to be sent from central Germany all the way to the Dutch East Indies to be tested by illiterate naval captains on scorbutic sailors. However, Moellenbrok did isolate crystals of a labile salt which he described as the 'volatile spirit of scurvy-grass.' A brilliant approach which, with any other vitamin apart from ascorbic acid, would have

(a)

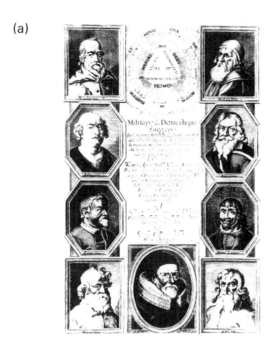

(b)

Of the Cure of the Scurvie.   165

shall finde there do farre exceede any that can be carried thither from England, and yet there is a good quantitie of Juice of Lemmons sent in each ship out of England by the great care of the Marchants, and intended onely for the reliefe of every poore man in his neede, which is an admirable comfort to poore men in that diseafe : also I finde we have many good things that heale the Scurvy well at land, but the Sea Chirurgeon shall do little good at Sea with them, neither will they indure. The ufe of the juyce of Lemmons is a precious medicine and well tried, being found and good, let it have the chiefe place, for it will deferve it, the ufe whereof is : It is to be taken each morning, two or three fpoonfuls, and faft after it two houres, & if you adde one fpoonfull of *Aquavitæ* thereto to a cold ftomack, it is the better. Alfo if you take a little thereof at night it is good to mixe therewith fome fugar, or to take of the fyrup thereof is not amiffe. Further note it is good to be put into each purge you give in that difeafe. Some Chirurgeons alfo give of this juice daily to the men in health as a prefervative, which courfe is good if they have ftore, otherwife it were beft to keep it for need. I dare not write how good a fauce it is at meat, leaft the chiefe in the ships wafte it in the great Cabins to fave vineger. In want where-

The Marchants are for Seamen.

Land medicines for the Scurvy bad Sea medicine.

The juice of Lemmons a good prefervative.

Plate 3.2 — Extracts from John Woodall's book *Military and domestique surgery*, published in 1617, which contains a chapter on the cure of scurvy. (a) The beautifully ornate frontispiece. (b) A description of the value of lemon juice for the cure of scurvy.

worked well. A more successful outcome might have advanced nutritional science by two and a half centuries. It was just bad luck that he was working with the most unstable of the vitamins.

An animal model for the study of scurvy

It was only in 1907 that the Danes, Holst and Frolich, noticed that it was possible to produce the signs of scurvy in the guinea pig. With such an animal model, rapid progress in the understanding of vitamin C nutrition was at last possible, leading to the final isolation of ascorbic acid by Szent-Gyorgyi, for which he got the Nobel Prize. In fact, like many findings in science, there was a certain amount of serendipity involved. Szent-Gyorgyi's wife gave him an inedible meal and, instead of putting it down the WC when she wasn't looking, he took it to his laboratory and found that it was very rich in vitamin C. His wife had put a lot of paprika in it — Hungarian red pepper — which is a good source of vitamin C. So, within days, he had crystals and most of the story of ascorbic acid was solved.

Discoveries in nutrition by great women scientists

Dr Cicely Williams (1893–, Plate 3.3) made, in 1931, the extremely important observation that a most devastating disease of the Third World called **kwashiorkor**, which mainly affected young children, was primarily protein deficiency (although we now know that a deficiency of energy also plays a part). Dr Williams gained the confidence of mothers in Ghana by running 'well baby clinics' to which mothers were encouraged to bring their infants to be admired. So mothers brought their infants even when they were believed to be in good health, and in this way early signs of illness could be detected. This approach was innovative, as previously mothers had only brought their infants in when they were near to death and very little could be done for them. Having gained the mothers' confidence, it was possible, when infants did die, to undertake post-mortems. Those that died had fatty livers, a sign that Dr Williams knew was not associated with infantile pellagra, which was the previous diagnosis of kwashiorkor (skin rash is common to both pellagra and kwashiorkor).

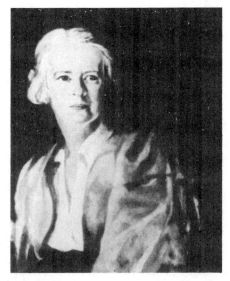

Plate 3.3 — Dr Cicely Williams (1893 –) named and described the devastating Third World disease called kwashiorkor. Two books have been written about her heroism as a prisoner of war during World War II, which are a testimony to a very remarkable lady.

The result was that the Colonial Medical Service dismissed Dr Williams, as there were so few infants coming into the hospital. It was assumed that she couldn't be bothered to admit infants but, in fact, she was so successful at curing early illnesses, that few infants became ill enough to warrant hospital treatment. She was transferred to the Far East and during World War II was taken prisoner by the Japanese. Immediately after the war, when the World Health Organization (United Nations) was set up, she was put in charge of maternity and child welfare and given a beautiful office in Geneva which she rarely used, as she spent so much time in the Third World advising mothers on nutrition. Two books have been written about her heroism during World War II, which are a testimony to a very remarkable lady.

Two other ladies have contributed greatly to nutrition: Dorothy Hodgkin and Dame Harriette Chick. Dorothy Hodgkin got her Nobel Prize for discovering the structure of vitamin B_{12}, which was the last vitamin to be elucidated. Dame Harriette Chick, who died five years ago at the age of 102, was one of the pioneers of vitamin research.

Observation: Inborn errors of metabolism
The discovery of inborn errors of metabolism was one of the very great advances in food and nutritional science, resulting from the work of Sir Archibald Garrod (1857–1936), who did not gain the recognition due to him. In 1909 he published a book called '*Inborn Errors of Metabolism*', of which there was a second edition in 1923. While 'fortune favours the prepared mind', there were three things which came together in Garrod's background which contributed to his genius. First, he was the son of a good biochemist, Sir Alfred Garrod (1819–1907), who was the first person to recognize the importance of uric acid in gout, so he knew about chemistry. Secondly, he was a children's doctor, so he frequently examined children in the presence of their sibs and parents. And, thirdly, he was a close friend of Bateson who was one of the rediscoverers of Mendel's work, so he knew about genetics.

That combination of knowledge produced his brilliant idea, that a person could carry genetic information leading to a missing or deranged enzyme (a single fault in an enzyme system) and therefore be born with a disease. Garrod was known as the 'Urine Doctor' at St Bartholomew's Hospital in London, because, in order to do his analyses, he had to collect gallons of urine from his patients. In those days large quantities of sample were necessary as chemical analyses were crude. However, after Garrod's death paper chromatography was introduced and analyses could be done even on a thimble-full of urine. Immediately, an enormous number of inborn errors of metabolism were discovered.

Lets take the example of phenylketonuria (PKU) to show how important inborn errors are in food and nutritional science.

As shown in Fig. 3.1, phenylalanine can be hydroxylated in the body to produce tyrosine. It is also metabolized by deamination to give phenylpyruvic acid (a keto acid), but this is toxic in high concentrations to the developing brain. So, if there is inhibition of the hyroxylase (block at point A in Fig. 3.1), phenylalanine and phenylpyruvic acid will accumulate and the latter will be excreted in the urine. There is a very simple test for this in the infant: just test the baby's nappy with ferric chloride and you get a green colour if phenylpyruvic acid is present.

Phenylketonuria affects about 1 in 30 000 of the population in the UK and is the cause

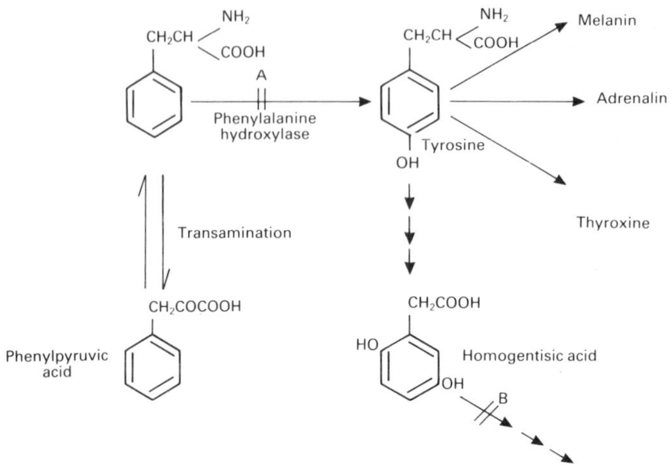

NH₂
CH₂CH COOH
A
Phenylalanine
hydroxylase

NH₂
CH₂CH COOH
Tyrosine
OH
Melanin
Adrenalin
Thyroxine

Transamination

CH₂COCOOH
Phenylpyruvic
acid

CH₂COOH
HO
Homogentisic acid
OH
B

Fig 3.1 — Metabolism of phenylalanine.

of about 0.5 to 1% of all patients in mental institutions, despite the fact that the mental consequences are totally preventable.

If a child is born with phenylketonuria and has a normal IQ when it is born, after about 20–25 months the child is an imbecile if the condition is untreated. When the cause of the imbecility in this disease was first discovered, there was much alarm, as it was thought that patients with PKU would have to be treated for the rest of their lives. We now know that this is not necessary, and that if treatment is early then any mental effects can be prevented.

Treatment is difficult but well worth while and involves putting the child on a diet low in phenylalanine, but not a diet free of phenylalanine, because it is an essential amino acid. As most proteins contain phenylalanine, it is usual to formulate a diet containing a mixture of synthetic amino acids (other than phenylalanine) or a specially prepared milk, with just sufficient phenylalanine for the requirement of the infant, without excess to form phenylpyruvic acid. Once the brain has developed, when the child is 8 – 10 years old, then he or she can revert to a normal diet, because only the developing brain is sensitive to high levels of phenylpyruvic acid.

The body converts tyrosine to melanin, to adrenalin, and also to thyroxine (see Fig. 3.1). **Albinism** is a block in the enzyme (tyrosinase) in the catabolism of tyrosine, such that melanin cannot form and therefore skin, eye and hair are unpigmented.

Another inborn error is alkaptonuria. Normally, tyrosine is metabolised to homogentisic acid, which has an extra hydroxyl group and is broken down further. The missing enzyme in alkaptonuria is at point B (see Fig. 3.1) and therefore in the alkaptonuric subject, homogentisic acid accumulates. This substance goes black in the urine on standing, since the urine becomes alkaline. When urine is allowed to stand, CO_2 is given off and urea, which is neutral, is broken down to ammonia, which causes the alkalinity. We know that this disease has existed since antiquity, as there are accounts of this phenomenon in the literature. In one account, a monk was dosed both outside and inside with ice-cold water to cool his internal organs as he was assumed to be inhabited by the devil. He is reported to have said, rather succinctly, that he didn't mind whether his urine went black on standing or not. Indeed, there are no symptoms to alkaptonuria, except an increased tendency to arthritis in old age, but it is a very interesting condition, for elucidation, of which Garrod should take the credit.

Few had realized how brilliant Garrod's work was. It is only now that certain Americans, who are catching up on the importance of his work, are seeking to write his life history. While the American, Beadle was working in Oxford in 1958, he was awarded the Nobel Prize for the 'one-gene-one-enzyme-hypothesis' (1945) and he had never heard of Garrod. He read Garrod's books and gave, in his Nobel lecture, credit to Garrod for having years earlier put forward the concept of a genetically-missing enzyme causing an error of metabolism.

Observation followed by experiment: Iodine and goitre

Sir Robert McCarrison (1878–1960) was a great nutritionist who spent most of his life in India, doing superb work under enormously difficult conditions. He went to India with the Medical Service just after the turn of the century. He made observations on the distribution of endemic goitre (which means that most people in the region had goitre, which is an enlargement of the thyroid gland, often caused by a lack of iodine in the diet). He noticed that, of nine villages which make up Gilgit in the foothills of the Himalayas, eight only had goitre, sometimes with cretinism. He did a classic experiment. He had noticed that the water supplies were different — the village without goitre had clear water coming down from a mountain spring, while the other eight had water polluted with sewage, passing from one village through the next with increasing incidence of goitre. He concentrated the two waters and fed them either to himself or to volunteers. Those that drank the polluted water got goitre (including himself), and those that took the clear water did not. His analysis of the two waters showed that the iodine contents of both were similar and of a normal level.

By this simple experiment he proved the existence of goitrogenic substances. We now know that there are two factors that contribute to endemic goitre. One is iodine deficiency in the diet or water, and the other is the presence in the diet of certain goitrogenic substances such as glucosinolates, which are particularly high in the *Brassica* family, such as cabbage and kale. These substances interfere with the uptake of iodine by the thyroid gland and inhibit the formation of the hormone thyroxine. Goitre has been shown in children who drank milk from cows fed on kale.

McCarrison was another person who did not receive the credit due to him. In his case it was because of the contemporary fashion in nutrition experiments. With the discovery of most of the vitamins, it was possible to conduct nutritional experiments with animals on purified, defined diets. Because of this, the use of experiments using whole diets was regarded as inferior. In fact, we now realize that both approaches are valid and their appropriateness depends on the circumstances. Although in human experimentation it is difficult to get the volunteers to eat synthetic, purified diets, the current trend in nutrition is to rely less heavily than before on results of experiments on lower animals. Although results from these experiments can be relevant to man, they cannot, because of the differences between species, predict the human state completely.

There is a lot of difference between countries in the prevalence of goitre. Wherever there is a low intake of iodine there is risk of goitre. Iodine deficiency produces not only goitre, however, but also cretinism — imbecility following growth inhibition *in utero*. I have seen cretins in hospitals in parts of the world as widespread as South America and Yugoslavia. Cretinism is a disease which is totally preventable by giving iodine to the pregnant mother and it is really horrible that this disease is allowed to occur, so that these imbeciles have to be put into mental hospitals, as once the condition is established, it is not reversible.

The solution to the problem of goitre and cretinism is quite straightforward and was adopted in Switzerland years ago. Switzerland had a long history of iodine deficiency. In 1755, the medically qualified Irish author, Oliver Goldsmith, travelled through Switzerland and was laughed at because he was thought to be deformed, as he did not have a goitre. Almost everyone in Switzerland had a goitre. Now there is no goitre in Switzerland because the Government has introduced the fortification of salt with iodine (potassium iodate). And various other countries have done this. In the UK, salt is not iodized — though in 1946 a survey in which I was involved showed goitre to be quite prevalent. In a village 13 miles from Oxford, called Hook Norton, goitre was endemic. The village baker had an enormous goitre and there was a case of cretinism.

As far as the iodization of salt is concerned, the law, in those countries that have introduced it, is that all salt readily available for sale should be iodized, within particular limits, with potassium iodate; but, that uniodized salt should be available at the same price for those who request it. No one has been forced to have iodized salt, as 1 person in 100 000 is sensitive to it, suffering blistering. This preservation of free choice is a very important principle in the nutrient fortification of foods. I want to illustrate it further with the case of fluorine.

Fluorine in food and water

I want it to be quite clear that my views are not those of the great majority of the medical profession. The medical and dental professions, because they know little about it, are in favour of adding fluorine to public water supplies. I happen to have worked with fluorine poisoning in a number of countries and was, until quite recently, President of the International Society for Fluoride Research, some of whose members support and others oppose fluoridation.

Plates 3.4 (a) and (b) show human bones from someone who died of fluoride poisoning compared with a normal person's bones. High levels of fluoride increase bone ossification (laying down of calciferous material) and can include tendons and ligaments. Darkening of the bone also occurs, although the reason for this is not clear. Plates 3.4(a) and 3.4(b) show that in the normal vertebra (A) and there is plenty of room for the spinal cord. In fluoride poisoning (vertebra (B)), the amount of bone is increased, so the spinal cord gets pinched because the space available for it is reduced. Where the nerves emerge from the spinal cord they also get pinched, causing paralysis. This is illustrated in Plate 3.4 (b) by the loosely rolled piece of paper, which shows a much smaller diameter in (B) than in (A).

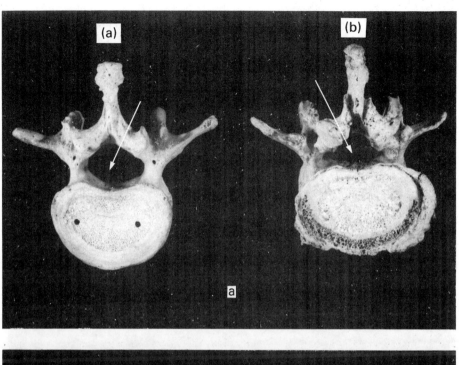

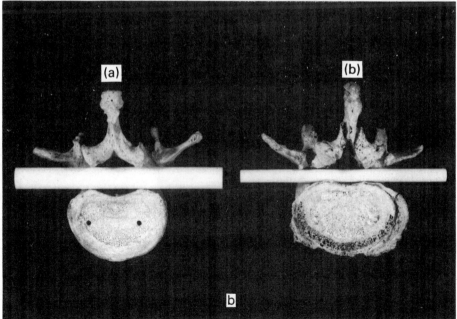

Plate 3.4 — A lumbar vertebra from a person with fluorosis (b), compared with a normal vertebra (a). (NB: Ignore the holes in the normal vertebra that have been made to assemble the skeleton.) 3.4(a) The size of the vertebral canal (arrow) is very much reduced in (b) compared with (a). 3.4(b) Specimens as in Plate 3.4(a), but with loosely rolled paper to show the size of the intervertebral foramen, which carries a spinal nerve, reduced in (b) compared to (b).

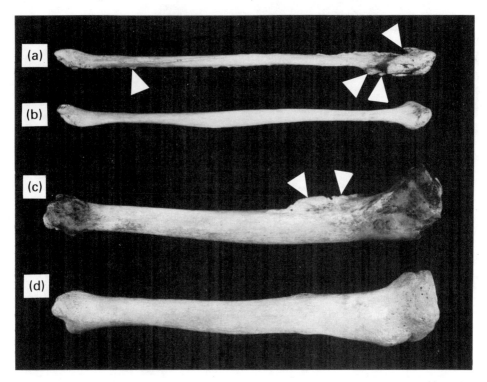

Plate 3.5 — Lower leg bones, tibia (A) and fibula (C), from a person with fluorosis compared with the equivalent bones from a normal person, (B) and (D). Note the increase in pigmentation of (A) and (C), and the calcification of tendons and ligaments, causing ossified protrusions (arrows).

The same applies to other bones. Plate 3.5 shows normal and abnormal human fibulas and tibias (lower leg bones), the abnormal with excessive amounts of bone and ossified tendons. A person suffering from very severe fluoride poisoning (fluorosis) may develop 'poker back' and the rigidity extends down the whole body such that you can pick them up by their head and their heels, as they are completely rigid. There are areas in Kenya which are notorious for fluoride poisoning and there is a tribe, the 'El Molo' on Lake Rudolf, who are dying out because of fluoride poisoning.

My main experience with fluorosis is in connection with India, particularly in the Punjab and near Hyderabad. In India there are well-defined areas of the country where fluorosis is endemic (Fig. 3.2). Small excesses of fluoride will show in the teeth: the first signs are chalky white patches on the teeth (at about 4 ppm fluoride in the water), and then these progress to mahogany staining of the teeth, which is permanent (Plate 3.6(a)). Plate 3.6(b) shows an Indian man with advanced fluorosis who cannot stand straight. Other men with fluorosis may not be able to bend their legs and so may have to shuffle along with sticks. The condition is rarer among women, because they drink less water.

The chances of getting fluoride poisoning in the UK are not great, but it is possible. Tea is particularly high in fluoride and can cause problems. I saw a case in our Oxford hospital — a 57-year-old carpenter who had developed fluoride poisoning. In Oxford the water is not fluoridated, but he drank daily 20 cups of tea without milk. Tea with milk leads to lower fluoride absorption because of the high calcium content of milk: calcium fluoride is very insoluble.

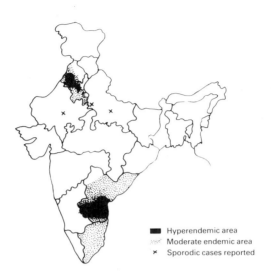

Fig 3.2 — Areas of endemic fluorosis in India.

Elderly people, especially old widows living in cottages alone, tend always to have a kettle on the boil. The one thing they have to look forward to is someone putting their head round the door to see if they are still alive. Then they will say, 'Do stop for a cup of tea — the kettle's is boiling.' This observation led us to experiment with the effects on fluoride concentration in water during prolonged boiling. The village in Oxfordshire where I live used to be supplied by an alkaline water that contained no calcium ions. The Fig. 3.3 shows the effects of concentrating this soft water and Oxford tap water by boiling. The latter is fairly hard. As you concentrate this, the fluoride content goes up only slightly, and stabilizes at about 10–20 ppm as the calcium fluoride precipitates in the 'fur' of the kettle. But the village water with no calcium ions behaves very differently: the fluoride can concentrate up to 1 000 ppm (1g per litre!).

Fluoride and public water supplies
Everyone has a right to a pure water supply, and mass medication by an authority to a water supply is, I think, unethical. The argument that adding fluorine to water is analogous to putting chlorine in water is not tenable, as chlorine is added to water to make it safe to drink, not because chlorine is good for you.

As I have said, mine is not a view commonly held in the medical profession, but I think that to allow an authority to add substances to the water supply just because it is thought that the population will benefit poses ethical questions which, in another context, could have sinister overtones. The following are some examples to illustrate my point.

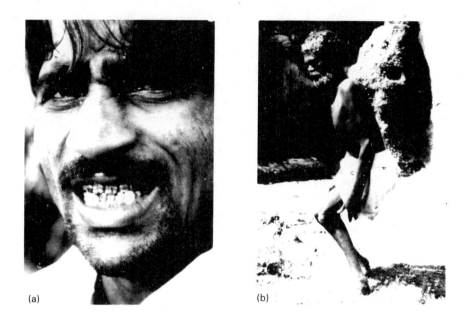

(a)   (b)

Plate 3.6 — Characteristic signs of fluorosis. (a) Permanent mahogany staining of the teeth. (b) This man is not able to stand upright.

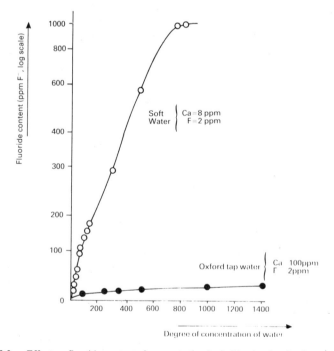

Fig 3.3 — Effect on fluoride content of concentrating by boiling hard and soft waters.

Mass medication of water
Population pressure in many parts of the world is now immense, and there is little doubt that this is the greatest problem facing mankind. It has been seriously suggested that authorities should put an oral contraceptive into the water supply and then anyone who is allowed by the state to have a baby is given the state anti-contraceptive.

Secondly, Arthur Koestler, a distinguished writer and the author of '*The ghost in the machine*' (1967), stated that we are all are slighly hypermanic and that if we calmed down a bit the world would be a happier place. Koestler seriously suggested that a mild tranquilizer could be put into the public water supply; football crowds would be more orderly!

The third example concerns the French prime minister, Mendez France. He instigated an anti-alcohol campaign and ordered lots of posters to be put up all over the Métro system. But there was very little evidence that they had any effect. Then his nutritional adviser suggested he could solve this problem by putting the drug 'Antabuse' in the water supply. This has no effect on a person until they take a little alcohol and then they are violently sick. This would also be unethical: Antabuse is used to treat alcoholics, but only if they **want** to be so treated.

Fortification of Foods
Certain foodstuffs, apart from salt are fortified by law in many countries. The classic example is margarine. This is a substitute (sometimes called an analogous food) for butter, but contains no vitamin A (retinol) or carotenoids and no vitamin D, whereas butter is very rich in these nutrients. As many groups of people rely heavily on butter for these nutrients, when margarine is substituted for butter it is important that these nutrients are also supplied. Therefore, by law, margarine has to be fortified by vitamins A and D within specific limits. Most preparations of cows' milk for infants have to be fortified with vitamin D and other nutrients. In these admirable examples, no one is forced to take the fortified substance, as there are alternatives; there is no alternative to water.

EXPERIMENTATION
The historical perspective of the development of experimentation in nutrition was dealt with to some extent in the Chapter 2. Discoveries in nutrition go hand in hand with other discoveries in science. Documentation of nutritional experiments started with digestion, but understanding of metabolism could not proceed until the gases were discovered following Robert Boyle. The use of purified diets was a similar milestone in nutritional science and much progress was made in our understanding because of them.

Purified diets: animal models
Vitamins were discovered in 1880 by Lunin (1853–1937), who was a young Russian scientist working in Switzerland. He put mice on a diet of the constituents of milk —

protein (casein), fat and carbohydrate (lactose), with an imitation of the salts of milk plus water — and he found the mice died in a few days. If he fed them fresh milk, they were still living happily at sixty days. However, the textbook discovery of vitamins is normally reported as that of Hopkins (1861–1947), who published a classic paper in 1912 describing an experiment in which he had repeated Lunin's experiment, but with rats. He obtained the same results and was awarded (together with Eijkman) the Nobel Prize. Eijkman (1858–1930) was a young medical officer in Java in the 1880s, who noticed that, in one of the prisons, when the inmates got beri-beri, the staff did not. He experimented with their diets and noticed that chickens fed with staff food did not get polyneuritis (the paralysis of beri-beri), whereas those fed with polished rice alone did. Eijkman's work led to the discovery of thiamin.

Purified diets: use with humans
In fact, the first experiments on purified diets were actually on humans rather than animals. The work was started by William Stark (1740–1770) in 1769 when he was a young doctor. He performed a classic experiment by putting himself on purified diets that made him very ill, which delighted him. To his purified diet he would then add extra foods to see their effects. For example, he might add honey, white bread, and sugar or olive oil; or honey alone; or just bread and sugar repeatedly, which gave him scurvy. After the twenty-fourth experiment he was very ill with scurvy and died miserably, at the age of 29. He had the distinction of the great Dr John Hunter doing the post-mortem. This was a brilliant approach, but with, alas, a fatal outcome.

Goldberger and pellagra
Immediately after Hopkins's work was published, McCollum (1879–1969) was able in 1913 to show the existence of fat- and water- soluble vitamins. That there was more than one water-soluble B vitamin was shown in 1926 by Goldberger (1874–1929). He was a genius. His parents, when he was five years old, had migrated from Hungary to the slums of New York, and Goldberger, as a child, ran errands for his father's little grocery store, educating himself from borrowed books from book stores when nobody was looking. He eventually obtained a scholarship, qualified in medicine and joined the US Public Health Service. (But like so many public health services today, they were not interested in advancing knowledge.) It was only by doing some of the most heroic experiments ever done that Goldberger proved that the disease **pellagra** was caused by a vitamin deficiency and was not an infection.

At the time, pellagra, rather like beri-beri, would break out in institutions and all the inmates would get ill at the same time and especially in the spring. Pellagra manifested as a skin rash and it was natural that everyone thought that it, like beri-beri, was an infection. In order to prove that it was not, Goldberger had the blood of pellagrins injected into himself and his gentile wife. Nevertheless, he was laughed at for maintaining that pellagra was a nutrient deficiency. So provoked was he that he even ingested pellagrous faeces to show that it was not an infection.

Then he did a classic experiment. With the consent of a prison governor and the inmates (each of whom was represented by his own attorney), he gave prisoners what he considered was a pellagrous diet. The deal was that if they ate this for six months, their sentences would be remitted. With only a few days to go, they developed pellagra. In fact, he actually produced riboflavin deficiency with scrotal dermatitis, but this was not known at the time. We now know that the skin rash of pellagra is limited to areas of the skin exposed to sunlight or other trauma. Nevertheless he had proved his point that the skin rash was due to the absence of something in the diet, rather than being due to an infection.

In his later years Goldberger claimed that pellagra was caused not merely by the deficiency of a pellagra-preventive vitamin (now known as nicotinic acid), but that an element from protein was also involved. The scientific community jeered at this and said he must be going senile. But he was right, because his main point was that milk was a very poor source of the pellagra preventive vitamin but very good in curing pellagra. We now know milk to be a very good source of the amino acid, tryptophan, which can be converted to nicotinic acid in the body. So, Goldberger was right!

The importance of ethics in human experimentation

I would like to stress an important point about experimentation on human beings. Goldberger's experiment which I have described was highly ethical. He got the informed consent of the prisoners and they knew exactly what the risks were. However, when you read in books on food and nutritional science of experiments on man pause to think whether those experiments should have been done or not, because frequently, alas, those done in the past were unethical. These days, before a paper will be accepted for publication, evidence that the experimental design has been scrutinized by an ethical committee needs to be submitted.

The work of Arild Hansen on essential fatty acid (EFA) deficiency serves to illustrate the point of unethical experimentation. At a Congress I organized in Oxford in 1957, Hansen produced his proof that EFAs were needed by humans. He work had been carried out on young children in his hospital in Texas. The children had been put on a fat-free diet and made severely ill with dermatitis. Hansen maintained that he had the informed consent of the mothers, who were all blacks of poor background. Informed consent meant nothing in this case, as any mother bringing her child to a distinguished hospital would sign any bit of paper: it is almost inconceivable that a distinguished paediatrician could deliberately make a child ill.

There was an even worse example during World War II concerning another American paediatrician. At the time it was debated whether riboflavin deficiency could produce cataract or not in man, although it could in monkeys. He told me that he had deliberately made two infants riboflavin deficient and had produced blindness by irreversible cataract. My contact with this person ceased forthwith.

A final example is the Vipeholm experiment (1954). This is, perhaps the classic experiment in dental medicine, but it should not have been conducted. Informed consent was obtained from the relatives of mental patients in a mental hospital at Vipeholm in Sweden. The patients were given a variety of diets, which included sugar in various forms, with or without a meal. The results were important, in that they showed that eating sticky forms of sugar between meals caused most dental caries, and the experiment is unique. But, the experiment ought never to have been done. The relatives of a mental patient are the worst people to give informed consent, as they are biased!

CONCLUSION

Advances in the food and nutritional sciences are made by observation and experiment. Observation includes epidemiology and compares diseases in different persons with what they eat. Experiments are ideally done on man, but great care must be taken to ensure they are ethical. If this is not practical, then experiments are done on lower animals, again with appropriate precautions. The treatments of previously lethal diseases (such as diabetus mellitus with insulin and pernicious anaemia with liver extract and then vitamin B_{12}) could not have been discovered without research using lower animals, in these cases, dogs. Similarly, the discovery and isolation of the different vitamins could not have been made without research in (mainly) rats and mice.

The triumphs of the last few years in the food and nutritional sciences have made our ignorance more precise. There are still many exciting discoveries to be made.

REFERENCES

Garrod, A. E. (1909) *Inborn errors of metabolism.* OUP, London. (2nd ed. (1923) Lancet, London.)

Goldberger, J., Waring C. H., and Tanner, W. F. (1923) *Pellagra prevention by diet among institutional inmates.* US Public Health Report. **38**, 2361–2368.

Gustafsson, B. E., Quensel, C.-E., Lanke, S. L. *et al.* (1954) The Vipeholm dental caries study. *Acta Odontologica Scandinavica.* **11**, 232–364.

Hansen, A. E., Adam, D. J. D., Wiese H. F. *et al.* (1958) Essential fatty acid deficiency in infants. In: Sinclair, H. M. (ed) *Essential fatty acids* Butterworth, London. pp 216–220.

Hopkins, F. G. (1912) Feeding experiments illustrating the importance of accessory–factors in normal dietaries. *Journal of Physiology.* **44**, 425–460.

Lind, J. (1753) *A Treatise of the scurvy.* Millar, London.

McCollum E. V. and Davis, M. (1913) The necessity of certain lipins in the diet during growth. *Journal of Biological Chemistry.* **15**, 167–175.

Moellenbrok, A. V. (1676) (Molimbrochius) *Cochlearia curiosa.* Cademan, London.

Stark, W. (1788) *The works of the late William Stark, M. D.* Johnson, London.

Williams, C. (1933) A nutritional disease of childhood associated with a maize diet. *Archives of Diseases of Childhood.* **8**, 423–433.

Woodall, J. (1617) *The Surgion's mate.* Griffin for Lisle, London.

4

Infant feeding

Ann Walker

Introduction

Human milk is a total food for the baby in the first few months of life. Normally, not even water needs to be given to the infant in addition to milk. Human milk fulfils two main functions. (a) It provides the infant with all of the nutrients required until weaning. (b) It protects the infant against infective agents. In addition, breastfeeding provides an invaluable social and emotional bond between the mother and child. Indeed, absence of this bond may be related to subsequent patterns of abnormal adult behaviour (e.g. aggressive tendencies) and even to the development of the brain tissue.

Few people, including leading nutritionists, would doubt that maternal milk constitutes the best food for the infant. However, before the advent of infant formulas (artificial milks), there was little alternative to a mother breastfeeding her infant, unless a wet nurse could be found. Even today, because of costs and unavailability of infant formulas in many of the poorer parts of the world, it is a sad fact that an infant's chances of survival there are remote if its mother cannot breastfeed it.

The energy and nutrients provided by human milk are required for growth and maintenance of the infant. Human babies use less for growth than most mammals as they are slow to mature: the infant is born with relatively immature kidney and liver. Indeed, myelination (formation of the sheath around the nerve axons) is not complete until about 3 years of age.

Requirements for energy and nutrients can be estimated from a knowledge of the composition of the infant at different ages. The composition has been determined by analysis of infants that have died by accident, but such data is scarce. Alternatively, requirements can be estimated from measurements of milk intake of healthy babies fed infant formulas. With a knowledge of the milk composition and the volume consumed, nutrient requirements can be estimated. It is considered unethical to carry out balance studies on babies, who are not in a position to volunteer for such work.

As far as is understood, human milk provides adequate amounts of all nutrients (except perhaps vitamin K in some cases) to satisfy the requirements of the child for up to the first 6 months of life. After that time, human milk will need to be supplemented with extra energy and iron.

In this chapter, after a discussion of trends in infant feeding, the compositions of human milk and cow's milk are compared. This serves to emphasize the important characteristics of human milk and the attention to modification that must be given to infant formulas based on cow's milk. Then the special disease protection of the baby afforded by human milk is discussed. Finally, attention is given to the weaning period.

INFANT FEEDING AND HEALTH

There is now a lot of evidence to show that infants that are breastfed have some advantages over those that are bottle-fed. One obvious difference is that the mortality rate is lower in infants who are breastfed, even in a country like the UK. The main contributing factors are (a) that human milk is very low in bacteria (the bacterial load) and (b) it contains antimicrobial factors).

In some developing countries, the mortality rate among bottle-fed infants may be very high indeed. Breastfed infants suffer fewer infections, in particular, gastroenteritis. In Britain there are fewer 'cot deaths' (sudden infant death) in breastfed babies. Many reasons have been suggested for this, but no one factor has emerged unequivocally. The suggestions include that some infants suffer an allergic reaction to cow's milk proteins.

A classical study of UK infants showed that the incidence of illness in general was less in breastfed infants. Similar results were obtained in Sweden and some other parts of the world. These studies were in countries with advanced sanitation, and therefore, it would be expected that differences would be even more acute in countries where sanitation was of a lower standard. In India, human milk is reported to protect low birth weight infants from infection: and reports from Brazil indicate that human milk can reduce infantile death due to respiratory infection; and diarrhoea.

In the UK, breastfeeding is strongly recommended by the government report *Present day practice in Infant Feeding* (DHSS, 1988):

> ...the Government Health Department should encourage all mothers to breastfeed their babies.

Regarding the timing of the introduction of solid food, the report is flexible. The overall recommendation on this point is:

> Very few infants will require solid foods before the age of three months but the majority should be offered a mixed diet not later than the age of 6 months.

Further clarification of this statement is made in the report:

> The length of time than an infant can fulfil its nutritional needs from human milk or infant formula alone varies considerably from baby to baby...... Because male babies are bigger than females, and grow more quickly, boys tend to be given mixed feeding sooner. Provided that the baby receives adequate nourishment and that due regard is paid to the development of feeding abilities, a flexible approach is desirable. ...... If the baby is reluctant to accept solids, and weight gain is satisfactory on milk alone, further diversification of the diet can be delayed until the infant accepts the food more readily."

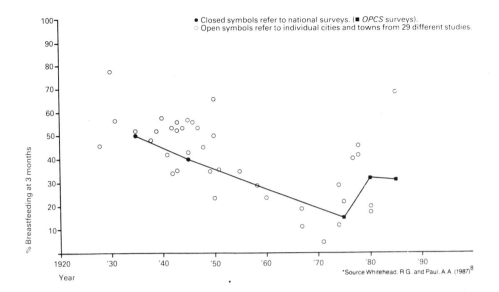

Fig. 4.1 — Proportion of mothers breastfeeding at 3 months, from 1920 to 1985 (England and Wales) DHSS (1988). Reproduced with permission from MRC Environmental Epidemiology Unit, Southampton, England.

Fig. 4.1 shows how rapidly breastfeeding declined in England and Wales the 1930s, with a nadir around the 1970s. This decline was coincident with the increased availability of good formula milks which closely mimicked the composition of human milk. In addition, the cultural tradition of breastfeeding declined, leaving a generation of women, whose own mothers had fed them on infant formula. Lack of confidence that breastfeeding provided sufficient nutrition for the infant abounded. Some of the reasons mothers gave for not breastfeeding are included in Table 4.1.

Table 4.1 — Common reasons for cessation of Breastfeeding

Given by mothers	Outside influences
Baby dissatisfied after feeding	Apathy of medical
Baby sucking poorly	profession
Depression	
Embarrassment	Breastfeeding no
Insufficient milk	longer part of
Neglect of husband	cultural heritage
Nipple damage	in UK
Restrictions on social life	
Tiredness	

In the early 1970s the medical profession did little to encourage breastfeeding, with mother and infant separated in hospitals and hospital routines making it very difficult for the infant to feed on demand, which is encouraged these days. Fortunately there has been a re-awakened interest in the feeding and nutrition of infants, together with a resurgence of breastfeeding (Fig. 4.1). This trend is particularly marked in the higher social classes (social classes 1 and 2 in Fig. 4.2).

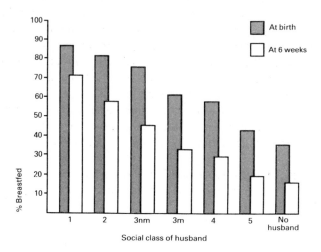

Fig. 4.2 — Proportions of infants put to the breast at birth and proportions of infants being breastfed at 6 weeks, by social class of husband (Great Britain, 1985). Classes range from Social class 1 (professional and managerial) to class 5 (unskilled); nm, non-manual; m, manual. (Source: DHSS, 1988.) Reproduced with permission of the Controller of Her Majesty's Stationery Office.

However, although the outlook seems positive for breastfeeding, the overall prevalence of breastfeeding is still less than 50% at 6 weeks of age. Even at birth, there is a high proportion of babies not put to the breast, at a stage when it is essential that they obtain the valuable supplies of colostrum (first milk — see below) from the mother. Table 4.2 shows the prevalence of breastfeeding in the years 1975, 1980 and 1985 in England and Wales of infants from birth to 9 months.

Table 4.2 — Breastfeeding in England and Wales
(as a percentage of sample studied)

Infant age	1975 (n=1544)	1980 (n=3755)	1985 (n=4671)
Neonate	51	67	65
1 week	42	58	57
2 weeks	35	54	53
6 weeks	24	42	40
4 months	13	27	26
6 months	9	23	22
9 months	—	12	12

Adapted from DHSS report (1988).

COMPARISON OF HUMAN MILK AND COW'S MILK

It must be remembered that the gastrointestinal tract and the kidneys of the new-born baby are relatively immature at birth, and this will affect digestion and absorption of nutrients, as well as the excretion of end-products of metabolism. The immature state of the baby means that its requirements for nutrients are very specific: enough nutrients are required for optimal growth of all tissues, but too much can be harmful. This is a very fundamental difference between infant nutrition and adult nutrition. For the infant, nutrient requirements are within a very narrow range, whereas for the adult, for most nutrients (except energy) a wide range of intakes are compatible with good health, as moderate excesses can be excreted.

Since cow's milk is normally used in infant formulas to substitute for human milk, it is important to note the compositional differences between the two milks, as they are very great. Giving unmodified cow's milk to newly born babies could seriously hinder their development.

There is another difference besides compositional differences: human milk contains a number of important antimicrobial agents, which are not present in cow's milk, or are present at a lower level.

Compositions of human milk and cow's milk

The composition of milk is most influenced by the course of lactation: the greatest differences being between colostrum (milk of the first few days of birth) and 'mature' milk (established milk supply). The composition of the milk of a mammal is related to the rate of growth and the changes in body composition of the young. Obvious differences in proximate composition of human milk and cow's milk can be seen in Table 4.3.

Table 4.3 — Proximate compositions of human milk and cow's milk

Component	Human	Cow's
Energy kJ/100 ml	290	273
Water g/100 ml	87.1	88.1
Protein g/100 ml	0.9	3.3
Fat g/100 ml	5.3	3.8
Carbohydrate g/100 ml	6.6	4.7

Adapted from Gurr, 1981.

Because of the ethical limitations on experimentation on human babies, we have more knowledge about nutritional requirements of young farm animals than of babies. However, it is known, that babies use a much larger proportion of their nutrient and energy requirements for maintenance (repair or tissues), whereas calves expend more in growth. The growth rate of offspring of various species is, indeed, related to the protein content of the milk as can be seen in Table 4.4.

Table 4.4 — Protein content of various milks in relation to growth of offspring

Animal	Time to double birth weight	Protein %
Calf	10 weeks	3.3
Pig	10–11 days	5.0
Rabbit	6 days	14.0
Human baby	20 weeks	0.9

Energy

Fat is the major source of energy in human milk. Another major source is the carbohydrate, lactose, which is broken down to glucose and galactose when digested and absorbed.

(a) Lactose

Lactose is not essential for the baby, in that galactose, which is necessary for the development of brain tissue, can be made in the body from glucose. However, lactose may perform a special function in maintaining gut homeostasis (see below) and in aiding the absorption of calcium. The lactose content of human milk is relatively high compared with cow's milk: lactose in human milk contributes about 40% of the total energy, while in cow's milk it supplies 29% of total energy.

If babies are given a dilute formula then they will take larger volumes, but not enough to compensate for the differences in energy density, so that their total energy intake will be less than that of babies receiving the correct formula. Energy density is therefore extremely important when considering the substitution of infant formulas for natural milk. It is also very important at weaning when weaning foods of low energy density can lead to malnutrition (see below).

(b) Fat

Human milk is high in the fatty acid, linoleic acid, compared to cow's milk (Fig. 4.3). In addition, human milk contains quite a lot of medium-chain fatty acids, but very little below C_{10}.

Fat from cow's milk is poorly absorbed by infants, in contrast to human milk fat. This is partly due to the poor solubility of the free long-chain saturated fatty acids derived from cow's milk during digestion. Fat absorption from human milk may be aided by two further factors:

(a) Human milk contains a high level of the amino acid taurine, which conjugates with bile salts. Bile salts are sodium salts of glycocholic or taurocholic acids, which contain glycine and taurine respectively. In formula-fed babies, sodium glycocholate predominates, which is not as efficient in forming emulsions of fat and water as sodium taurocholate.

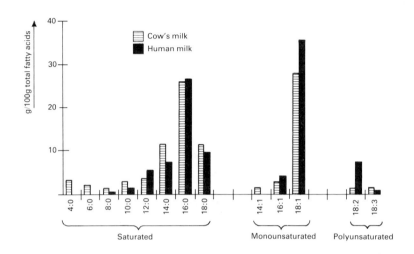

Fig. 4.3 — Fatty acid compositions of human milk and cow's milk.

(b) There is a low level of calcium in human milk. In cow's milk, the longer chain
    saturated fatty acids tend to form insoluble and poorly absorbed soaps with
    calcium.

   Human milk is rich in lipase, which rapidly liberates free fatty acids, even if the
milk is stored in the refrigerator. The liberation of fatty acids from the glycerol moiety
is at the 1 and 3 positions. Human digestive lipase has a similar action. Saturated
fatty acids esterified into triacylglycerols in human milk are present in the 2
position, and because this bond is normally not broken during digestion, saturated fatty
acids are therefore absorbed as the monoacylglycerol. In cow's milk, the saturated
fatty acid, palmitic acid, is present in the triacylglycerols in 1 and 3 positions and,
therefore, is liberated and free to form insoluble soaps with calcium. This leads to the
loss of fat and calcium in the faeces.
   Human milk has a very high level of cholesterol (12–25 mg cholesterol per 100
g). The reason for this is not known, but it has been suggested that it is to 'prime' the
metabolic routes against the future intake of dietary cholesterol.

(c) Protein
Not only is the amount of protein in human milk very different (much lower) than in
cow's milk, but also its composition differed very considerably from that in cow's milk.

Human milk has a much lower proportion of casein (see Fig. 4.4), which means that by the action of rennin, the milk forms a soft, flocculent, easily digested curd in the infant's stomach. Cow's milk (especially if it is unprocessed), because of its high casein content, forms a large firm curd by the action of rennin and is, therefore, less easily digested by the infant.

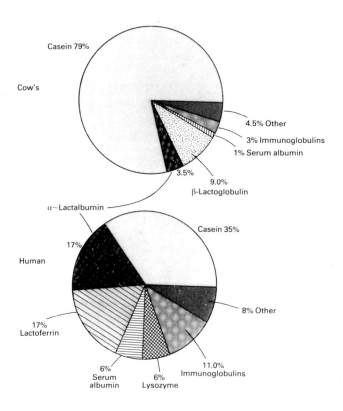

Fig. 4.4 — Protein compositions of human milk and cow's milk.

Whey proteins dominate in human milk (Fig. 4.4), and the most striking difference between human milk and cow's milk is the absence of β-lactoglobulin in human milk, while it is the predominant protein in the whey of cow's milk. The presence of β-lactoglobulin in cow's milk may account for allergy reactions to cow's milk, which develop in some infants.

If a baby were fed solely on cow's milk, to meet its energy requirements, it would take in about three times as much protein as it needs. This extra protein would have to be broken down, and the immaturity of the liver and kidneys are such that a rise in the blood free amino acids and urea will result. There is evidence that a high concentration of amino acids in the blood can cause damage to nervous tissue, especially in infants of low birth weight, whose kidneys are even more immature. High levels of tyrosine, in particular, may lead to lower intelligence. It is important, therefore, that infants are not fed high protein diets in the first few months of life.

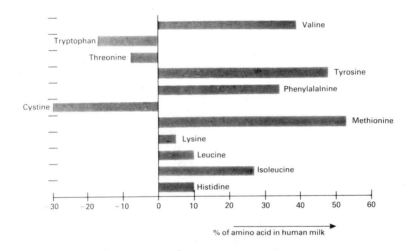

Fig. 4.5 — The amino acid profile of cow's milk compared with human milk. Percentage of individual amino acids in human milk compared with cow's milk. (Values for amino acids in cow's milk = 100.)

Another reason for raised levels of urea and free amino acids when infants are fed on cow's milk is the difference in the amino acid patterns of the proteins of the two milks (see Fig. 4. 5), owing to the differences in casein content. Human milk protein has an amino acid composition fitted for the requirements of the new-born baby. Other proteins with sub-optimal patterns of amino acids will have a deficiency of one or more amino acids, and an excess of others, resulting in an increased concentration in the blood of urea, ammonia and some amino acids.

The major difference between the amino acid patterns of the two types of milk is the higher ratio of cystine:methionine in human milk, which reflects the higher proportion of whey proteins that have a ratio of cystine:methionine about 10 times greater than casein. In fact, human milk has the highest cystine:methionine ratio of all sources of animal protein, being relatively rich in cystine. As far as the nutrition of the infant is concerned, the problem comes, because, although cystine can be readily synthesized from methionine in adults, the enzymes involved (cystathionine synthase and cystathionase) are absent or limiting in babies. Hence cystine is an essential amino acid in the newborn. It is converted into taurine, which is thought to be involved in the growth of the brain tissue. The brain is at its maximum growth in early infancy.

(d) Minerals
The differences in the mineral contents of human and cow's milk can be seen in
Table 4.5.

Table 4.5 — Minerals in human milk and cow's milk (mg/100 ml)

	Human	Cow's
Major minerals		
Sodium	15	50
Potasium	55	150
Calcium	33	120
Magnesium	3	12
Chlorine	43	95
Phosphorous	15	95
Ca:P ratio	2.2	1.3
Some minor minerals		
Iron	70	50
Zinc	290	350
Copper	39	20
Manganese	1.2	3
Chromium	0.6	1

Adapted from Gurr, 1981.

New-born infants have a relatively poor capacity to excrete excess salt compared
with adults. Not only is their glomerular filtration rate (rate of passage of blood
through kidney) lower, but also there is an inability of the renal tubules (responsible for
reabsorption of nutrients when the blood is filtered by the kidney) to reject sodium.
Thus the high sodium concentration of cow's milk can result in high blood sodium
levels and clinical problems such as dehydration (hypernatraemia). Homeostatic
disturbances in salt balance of this kind are more likely to occur in conditions of
diarrhoea, fever and low water intake, as sometimes happens when infants are fed
infant formulas that are too concentrated. This leads to gastroenteritis, which gives even
greater water loss, causing dehydration and hypernatraemia. Fortunately, now that
the problem is understood better, hypernatraemia is uncommon. As well as the problem
of hypernatraemia, there is also evidence from animal experiments, that an excessive
sodium intake in early life may lead to hypertension (high blood pressure) later.
  Of particular importance is the higher concentration of sodium and phosphorus and
the very low ratio of calcium:phosphorus in cow's milk compared with human milk.
Calcium is better absorbed by the baby from human milk than from cows' milk. This
difference may be related to the composition of the milk fat (see above), or to the higher
ratio of Ca:P. Excessive phosphorus can result in the formation of insoluble
calcium phosphates, which prevent the absorption of calcium. Hypocalcaemia may
result in the condition of neonatal tetany (twitching of limb muscles), which occurs
more often in formula-fed than in breastfed infants.

A child born at term (after 9 months) carries quite a high store of some minerals, including iron, zinc and copper. The milks of nearly all mammals have a low content of iron, which is bound to lactoferrin, an antimicrobial protein. Iron deficiency anaemia is rare in breastfed infants, but is more common in those fed infant formulas. This difference has been attributed to a higher bioavailability of iron from human milk, but the reasons for this are not understood. Zinc is relatively abundant in human milk: although cow's milk has a higher content, this is poorly absorbed.

(e) Vitamins
The vitamin content of human milk and cow's milk are given in Table 4.6.

Table 4.6 — Some vitamins in human milk and cow's milk (per 100 ml)

Vitamin	Human	Cow's
Water-soluble		
B_{12} µg	<0.01	0.3
C mg	3.8	2.0
Folic acid µg	5	5
Niacin µg	230	80
Riboflavin µg	30	190
Thiamin µg	5.9	40
Fat-soluble		
A µg	60	27–36
D µg	0.06	0.02
E µg	350	90

Adapted from Gurr, 1981.

In fact, not a great deal is known about the infant's requirements for vitamins. Except for nicotinic acid (niacin), the concentration of all vitamins of the B complex are higher in cow's milk than in human milk. Whereas most of these substances can be detected as the free vitamin, at least two of them, folic acid and vitamin B_{12}, are firmly bound to specific binding proteins. As for the fat-soluble vitamins, vitamin D may be mostly present in human milk in a water-soluble form, which has only been appreciated fairly recently.

As for vitamin K, a lack of this causes haemorrhagic disease of the newborn, and this is more common in breastfed babies than in bottle-fed ones. It is a transient disease at 2–6 days of life. There is a low prothrombin level and this leads to haemorrhage, with a raised level of pigments, causing jaundice which is distressing to the parents. Vitamin K is normally produced in the microflora of the gut, and once these become established then the problem rights itself. The illness can be readily cured by the administration of vitamin K.

Antimicrobial Factors

Apart from the 'ideal' composition of human milk for the baby, breastfeeding also confers greater protection for the child against infection from pathogenic organisms. One of the main features of human milk is that the bacterial count is very low compared to cow's milk: the latter needs to be collected and stored, so there is ample opportunity for contamination. Cow's milk has to be sterilized or pasteurized before use to make it safe for consumption, and this process will have the adverse effects of removing antimicrobial factors present. Therefore, a child fed on infant formulas derived from cow's milk will obtain no immune factors. Successful formula feeding relies on strict hygiene control, with sterilization of apparatus and feed being of the utmost importance.

Specific antimicrobial factors

Different strategies are employed by the human and the cow for the immunological protection of the newborn (Table 4.7). Whereas, in humans, the principal route of transfer of passive immunity is the transmission of immunoglobulins (IgG) from the mother across the placenta to the foetus, the cow relies principally on the transfer of immunoglobulins from colostrum into the newborn's circulation after birth, at a time when the gut is permeable to intact protein molecules. In humans, less than 50% of the immune factors are passed to the infant in the colostrum. Indeed, the chief immunoglobulin in human milk is not intended for absorption in this manner. This is secretory IgA. It is not absorbed and is active throughout the gut. Its function is:

(a) to neutralize toxins or viruses
(b) to inhibit bacterial adhesion to the intestinal wall
(c) to prevent the absorption of food antigens
(d) to suppress bacterial growth
(e) to aid phagocytosis by bringing about the attachment
      of bacteria to macrophages.

Table 4.7 — Immune factors in human milk and cow's milk

Factor	Human	Cow's
B_{12} or folic acid binding factors	++++	++++
Immunoglobulins		
IgA	++++	+
IgG	+	++++
Lactoferrin	++++	+++
Lactoperoxidase	+	++++
Lymphocytes	++	na
Lysozyme	++++	+
Macrophages	++++	++++

na, not available
Adapted from Packard, 1982.

Non-specific antimicrobial factors

Lysozyme is an enzyme that degrades bacterial cell walls in general. There is a high content of it in human milk. Lactoferrin is the second most abundant whey protein in human milk. It binds iron strongly, thus making it unavailable to bacteria such as pathogenic coliform organisms, which have high metabolic requirements for this metal.

Other antimicrobial factors include the vitamin-binding proteins for vitamin B_{12} and folic acid, which bind these vitamins in tight complexes, making them unavailable for the growth of pathogenic bacteria in the gut, which also have a requirement for these nutrients.

Milk also contains some whole cells whose normal function in the body is to act as part of the body's defence against pathogenic organisms. These are lymphocytes (white blood cells) and macrophages. The latter produce lactoferrin and lysozyme, and are capable of engulfing pathogenic bacteria and destroying them.

There are two other factors which may contribute to the fight against invading environmental organisms:

(a)   The antimicrobial activity of fatty acids, particularly medium-chain saturated and long-chain unsaturated ones.

(b)   the 'Bifidus' factor. Lactose is readily digested by the baby, but the high amount in human milk means that a small amount escapes digestion. This may be fermented by bacteria in the colon to lactic acid and volatile fatty acids. This fermentation, in conjunction with the low buffering capacity of human milk, results in a lowering of colon pH, and is in part responsible for suppressing the growth of pathogenic organisms like *Echerichia coli*, *Shigella* and protozoa in breastfed babies. In this environment, colonization by *Bifidobacterium* and *Lactobacillus* occurs. Bifido bacteria constitute 99% of the total flora of breastfed babies, but are not present in the flora of bottle-fed babies. It has been suggested that the presence of the Bifido bacteria themselves may be protective against infection.

Factors affecting the nutrient content of human milk

Ten days after birth, human milk is termed mature and does not change appreciably in composition after that, although the baby needs to adjust its intake to the changing requirements as it gets older. Fig. 4.6 shows how this intake increases, but only up to a maximum, which is the maximum which can be produced by the mother.

Human milk composition varies only slightly, depending on the stage of lactation, time of day, the method by which the sample is taken, and the nutritional status of the mother. The biggest change in composition is due to stage in lactation: colostrum versus mature milk.

Colostrum versus mature milk

In the first five days or so of lactation, the milk is known as colostrum, and has a very different composition from mature milk (Table 4.8). It is a clearer fluid than mature milk, and is mainly composed of protein, the level of which declines rapidly during the first week. The major change in composition is the decrease in the proportion of

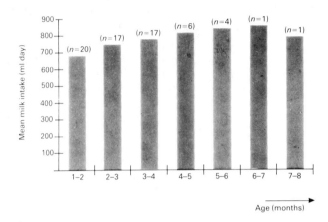

Fig. 4.6 — Milk intakes of fully breastfed female babies (ml/day) in Cambridge.

Table 4.8 — Composition of human colostrum compared with mature human milk
(g/100 ml)

Component	Colostrum	Mature Milk
Fat	2.9	4.2
Lactose	5.3	7.0
Total protein	10	1.1
Casein	1.6	0.5
Whey proteins	1.1	0.3
IgA	5.4	0.2
IgG	0.1	0.01
Lactoferrin	1.4	0.2

antimicrobial protein: whereas about 65% of the protein of colostrum is secretory IgA and lactoferrin, mature milk has less than 20% of the protein as antimicrobial protein. In addition, colostrum also contains a greater number of defensive cells (lymphocytes and macrophages) than mature milk.

Nutrient variations in mature milk
In any particular feed of mature milk, the effect of the stage of a feed on the composition of milk is mainly a change in the fat content. Thus 4–5 times as much fat and 1.5 times as much protein can be present in mature milk at the end of a feed compared with that at the beginning.

Although the fatty acid content of mature milk can vary with diet, there are not the day-to-day variations which are found with fat content. Linoleic acid, which is the principal essential fatty acid, originates from the diet, as it cannot be synthesized by animals. It is not surprising, therefore, that the linoleic acid content is considerably influenced by diet.

The vitamin content can vary also with the nutritional status of the woman. On the whole, the influence of malnutrition is not very great on the protein content and volume of milk, although starvation or severe malnutrition of the mother will result in reduced levels of both of these.

Human milk banks

Human milk collected for milk banks, for use with premature and 'at risk' infants, will contain a high bacterial count. It is recommended that human milk in milk banks is pasteurized, particularly now that there is evidence that HIV (the virus causing the AIDS syndrome) can be passed to babies through human milk. Pasteurization will inactivate all immune bodies and defensive cells, so that an infant fed such milk will not benefit in this respect; but it will still be able to have the benefit of human milk's ideal composition for babies.

Processing will affect the nutrient content of milk, particularly the content of vitamins. Some mothers express milk for their own babies, and this need not be pasteurized (assuming they are not HIV carriers) and can be stored frozen. Even in frozen storage there would be changes, as some of the lymphocytes are destroyed by freezing. Fresh human milk, frozen and stored at -70°C still retains antimicrobial activity, but storage at higher temperatures leads to gradual loss of this activity.

As far as heat treatment is concerned, pasteurization causes some loss of water-soluble vitamins (25% of vitamin C will be lost) and protective factors are damaged. IgA is well preserved under mild pasteurizing conditions (62.5°C for 30 min), but destroyed progressively if heating is more severe. Some losses of other non-specific antimicrobial agents will occur and lymphocytes and macrophages are destroyed.

INFANT FORMULAS

Any substitute for human milk can only be as good as current technology allows. (Packard, 1982)

Only in the present century have technological developments in dairying, food manufacturing, infant nutrition, environmental hygiene and sanitation, and a rise in socioeconomic and educational levels made widespread formula feeding of human babies practicable for the majority of people in the industrializ ed countries. Even so, no infant formula exactly meets the infant's changing requirements during the first months of life.

A recommended composition of a modern infant formula is given in Table 4.9. The starting material for most infant formulas is cow's milk. As explained above this is most unsuitable in its unmodified form: it is particularly important to reduce the protein concentration and the mineral load, especially sodium.

Table 4.9 — Recommended composition of a formula milk

Energy	270–315 kJ/100 ml
Protein	1.2–1.9 g/100 ml
Casein:whey ratio	20:80
Lactose	5–8 g/100 ml
Fat	3–5 g/100 ml
of which polyunsaturates	8–10% by weight

Adapted from Gurr, 1981.

The earliest and simplest approach was to add extra carbohydrate (preferably lactose) and dilute cow's milk to reduce the concentration of protein, fat and minerals per unit of energy intake. The disadvantage to this approach is that the amount of carbohydrate that is required to achieve the desirable reduction in mineral and protein concentration is about 10 g/100 ml, which is much more than is present in human milk. 'If this were added as lactose, then there would be danger of lactose malabsorption and fermentation in the colon, leading to diarrhoea. The addition of sucrose would not be suitable, as this may predispose infants to dental caries, and (possibly) obesity.

Another early attempt at modifying cow's milk was (in additition to those mentioned above) to change the fat source, as the fat from cow's milk is not well digested. This was called SMA (scientific milk adaption) and involved substituting the butter fat with mixtures of animal and vegetable fats or vegetable oils. There was, in fact a threefold aim to the production of SMA from cow's milk base:

(a)   Improved fat absorption.

(b)   Improved calcium absorption — the poor absorption of the fat of cow's milk influences the amount of calcium absorbed and this can lead to hypocalcaemia and tetany in the neonate.

(c)   Increase in the proportion of polyunsaturated fatty acids (PUFA) to bring them more into line with PUFA content of human milk.

A study by Dr Elsie Widdowson, of a number of infant formulas sold in Europe in the early 1970s, revealed that as far as the unsaturated fatty acids were concerned, all except two of the formulas had far more fat as linoleic acid than human milk!

Recently, modified milks have become available in which not only are the fats modified, and the carbohydrate and protein contents adjusted, but the whey:casein ratio has been changed by the use of demineralized whey, to provide an amino acid pattern more closely resembling the human pattern (Table 4.10). Even so, these infant formulas are but poor imitations of human milk, as β-lactoglobulin is present and the other cow's milk proteins and there are no anti-infective agents.

Table 4.10 — Comparison of composition of human milk, cow's milk and formula
milks (per 100 ml: formula at recommended dilution)

	Human	Cow's	Formula Gold Cap SMA a	Premium b
Energy, kJ	290	273	273	273
Protein, g	1.3	3.3	1.5	1.8
Casein:whey protein ratio	35:63	79:21	40:60	33:66
Fat, g	4.1	5.3	3.6	3.4
Fat source	Human	Cow	Animal + Veg.	Butterfat + Veg.
Lactose, g	7.2	4.7	7.2	6.9
Renal solute load, mOsm	8.5	33	9.1	11.3
Sodium, mmol	0.6	2	0.65	1.0

a, Wyeths; b, Cow & Gate; mOsm, milliosmoles – a measure of osmotic pressure.
Adapted from Francis, 1981.

Cow's milk whey is a by-product of the cheese-making industry, and by using demineralized whey, the mineral content of the modified milks can be decreased. Thus, by mixing appropriate amounts of skim-milk (to provide casein) and demineralized whey (to provide whey proteins and lactose) a casein:whey protein ratio similar to that in human milk can be achieved. The composition is completed by adding more lactose, minerals, vitamins and fat and the product is homogenized and spray-dried. Although it is only a crude imitation of human milk, it is nearer to the amino acid content of human milk, and appears to promote better growth in low birth weight infants than earlier formulas did.

Apart from the levels of the main sources of energy and protein, there is still a lot of controversy over the optimal levels of minerals and vitamins to add to infant formulas. While the composition of human milk remains as the yardstick, some nutritionists have argued that nature can be improved upon as far as mineral content is concerned. In particular, there is controversy over the levels of iron, as it has been suggested that the level of iron in human milk is too low and that breastfed infants are at risk of anaemia. In addition, there is still some debate about the form in which iron should be added, as not all forms are biologically available. On the one hand, the infant needs to be supplied with an adequate level of 'available' iron, but on the other hand, too great a quantity of iron may saturate the lactoferrin and thus eliminate its antimicrobial properties. This uncertainty has resulted in a widely varying range of iron levels being added by manufacturers to infant formulas. The top of this range is several fold in excess of that in human milk.

With all infant formulas it is essential that they are made up correctly. Most manufacturers provide instructions and a scoop for the measurement of powder. Incorrect dilution can lead to :

— over-concentrated formulaes :   this can cause obesity or even dehydration;

— under-diluted formulaes :   this is more likely to happen in the Third World, where a mother finds feeding the child by bottle too expensive and cuts down on solids

In the Third World, water supplies are often not potable, bottles not sterilized and consequently feeds are unhygienically prepared. An additional problem is that a lack of education means that mothers will not be able to understand formula preparation instructions. A combination of these factors leads to diarrhoea and malnutrition in infants that are formula fed, and for these reasons bottle feeding should not be encouraged in Third World countries. Indeed, companies which market these products are now discouraged from advertising their products to the general public in these countries.

Economics of formula feeding

Studies in the Third World show that it costs about 40% more for a mother to bottle-feed her baby than to breastfeed the child herself and to bear the cost of the extra food that she requires for this. For formula feeding there is also the cost of the bottles, sterilization and wastage. In some poor countries, formula for an infant may cost as much as 1/4–1/3 of the entire wages of a household.

Another aspect which may be considered from an economic point of view is that, while a mother is lactating, the chances of her becoming pregnant again are reduced because ovulation is suppressed. This natural method of birth control may have a considerable effect in some parts of the Third World where the rate of population increase is high.

THE WEANING PERIOD

Weaning is the introduction of solids. Normally, it coincides with the cutting of teeth and the child sitting up. Solid foods are firstly introduced into the diet as a sloppy gruel along with milk and then progressively given to the child in a more solid consistency as it gets older, finally replacing milk altogether, when weaning is complete. There can be adverse effects from the introduction of solids into the diet at too early an age. Apart from risks of the development of allergy in the newly born, early weaning can lead to the intake of too much energy and therefore result in obesity, or (and this is the case in many Third World countries) the semi-solid food prepared from starchy staples is so low in energy density that it may fill up the baby, reducing demand for milk and leading to protein-energy malnutrition. Traditional weaning foods may be only one third of the energy density of human milk.

By 1 year of age, bottle feeding should be discontinued and normally breastfeeding also, although longer breastfeeding in some parts of the Third World can provide the infant with an important supplement of protein, vitamins and energy.

Weaning is a very vulnerable time of human life. In the Third World, it is known that the incidence of diarrhoea in infants is low while the child is being breastfed, but during weaning it is so common that it has become known as the 'weaning disease'. There is a high infant mortality due to this. Infantile diarrhoea is due to the use of non-potable water being used to make up starchy gruels for the child. Often these are kept for as long as a day and fed to the child at intervals for convenience. The combination of the low energy density of the traditional starchy weaning food and diarrhoea can easily precipitate malnutrition.

Late weaning of the child (around 2 years of age) may be a common practice in some parts of the world, and it is then that the introduction of weaning foods containing milk powder can be a problem because of the lactose content. In some parts of the world, people cannot fully digest lactose into adult life (after the weaning period the secretion of lactase falls very quickly in these individuals). The problem will normally become evident at about 2 years of age. The lack of ability to digest lactose is caused by the lack of the enzyme lactase into adult life, and the inability to deal with lactose under these circumstances is termed lactose intolerance.

CONCLUSION

Breast milk has the following advantages when used for infant feeding:

(a) It is a major preventive measure, available throughout the world, which will markedly reduce infant mortality and disease.

(b) It meets the nutritional needs of the infant, particularly in respect of its mineral concentration, its amino acid composition and its fat digestibility.

(c) It provides a strong social bond between infant and mother.

(d) It is low cost.

There is still a place, and probably always will be, for infant formulas, when mothers are just not able to breastfeed, although the weight of evidence suggests that breastfeeding is the ideal to be sought wherever possible. The objective in the formulation of infant formulas should be to mimic human milk as closely as possible.

REFERENCES

DHSS (Department of Health and Social Security) (1988) *Present day practice in infant feeding: Third Report.* Report on Health and Social Subjects No. 32. HMSO, London.

Francis, D. E. M. (1981) Infant nutrition. In: Birch G. G., and Parker K. J., eds *Food and Health: Science and Technology.* Applied Science Publishers Ltd. London,

Gurr, M. I. (1981) Review of the progress of dairy science: human and artificial milks for infant feeding. *Journal of Dairy Research* **48**, 519–554.

Packard, V.S. (1982) *Human milk and infant formula.* Academic Press, New York.

Poskitt, E. M. E. (1983) Infant feeding: a review. *Human Nutrition: Applied Nutrition,* **37A**, 271–286.

Walker, A.F. (1990) The contribution of weaning foods to protein-energy malnutrition. (To be published in *Nutrition Research Reviews.*)

Wharton, B (ed.) (1986) Food for the Weanling. Proceedings of a symposium on Feeding the Older Infant and Toddler. *Acta Paediatricia Scandinavica*, Supplement **323**. 1–102.

5

Nutrition of specific human groups

Hugh Sinclair

Introduction

Much nonsense about nutrition is written in popular books on the subject. Would-be authors come to my Institute near Oxford, interview me with a tape recorder and then go home and write a little book. A lot of money can be made from misinformation in such books, particularly those on slimming. One well-known writer of popular romance with a huge reputation wrote a book about honey. The statement in that book — 'If you were isolated on a desert island, honey is the

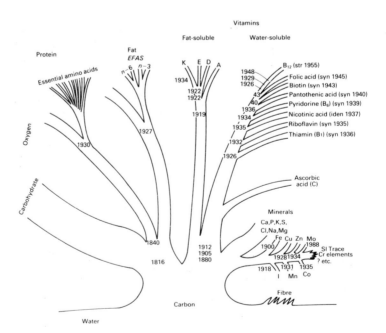

Fig. 5.1 — The Nutrient Tree: the evolution of our knowledge of ailments (energy-producing substances) and nutrients (essential amino acids, essential fatty acids, essential elements, vitamins). (EFA, essential fatty acid; iden, identified; str, structure; syn, synthesized.)

one thing you could live on indefinitely' — would make an intriguing subject for a Final Year degree examination reworded: 'If you were to eat nothing but honey what nutrient deficiency would you die of?'

Of the substances shown on the nutrient tree (Fig. 5.1), honey contains only carbohydrate and no vitamins. Lack of vitamin C would begin to give you scurvy in about 80 days (William Stark developed scurvy on only honey in a shorter time — see Chapter 4), but you would be dead before that, and not of protein deficiency because the protein supplies in the muscles would be used for a long period of time. It is debatable which would be more severe, energy or thiamin deficiency. It is more than likely that honey in such quantities would cause nausea, which would limit energy intake. Even if that were not so, with a high carbohydrate diet the requirements for thiamin would increase, as thiamin requirements are proportional to the percentage contribution to energy of carbohydrate in the diet; you would probably die of beri-beri.

HUMAN DIETS AND DIET-RELATED DISEASES

Humans are essentially vegetarian, like the great apes. Indeed, for the longest period of human history vegetarianism dominated. Man as a hunter/gatherer came later, as tools were necessary for hunting animals: humans are not well endowed with natural weapons such as claws or fangs to catch other animals. Once there were tools, man started to kill and eat beasts and even his own kind. Man became an agriculturalist and a pasturalist about 10 000 years ago; then famines started to occur from failure of crops.

The Ice Age about 50 000 years ago has provided us with the first evidence of nutritional disease: rickets. Perhaps it is not surprising that it should be this condition for which the earliest evidence persists, as the disease alters bone structure and, of course, bones are by far the most common relic of early man's inhabitation of the planet. Most of the rackitic bones discovered of this era belonged to women. The supposition is that they spent most of their time in caves, getting little of no sunlight, while the men were out hunting and making plenty of vitamin D.

There are a still a few hunter/gatherers in existence even today — such as the Kung bushman in North-West Botswana. These are very isolated and there is a ring around them of about 80 miles in diameter of desert. Despite their inaccessibility, they have been studied by investigators living with them, recording their eating and sociological habits. They are mainly vegetarian, although the men go out to hunt beasts, while the woman gather roots. Among these roots is one root which is very rich in linoleic acid — one of the essential fatty acids. This may contribute to their good health as, in general, they have very few diseases, apart from infections. They are long-lived, have no obesity and no dental caries, in fact none of the western diseases of affluence. However, the teeth are worn down by chewing roots.

There are many human ethnic groups in the world who have very different eating patterns. Some examples are:

— *Pastoralists*, e.g. Lapps, who eat raindeer; Iranian nomads with their sheep and goats; Tibetan nomads with yaks; African Tuareg with camels; Fulani and Masai with their cattle.
— *Slum and shanty town dwellers*, who are increasing in number.
— *Rich people* with their western diseases.

A study of the patterns of disease among different human groups is called epidemiology, which is a branch of observation, discussed in Chapter 3.

Epidemiology
This includes a study of the geographical distribution of disease and of the diets of the persons living in different localities or migrating from one to another. For instance, most western diseases are rare in Japan (though now increasing with alteration of diet), but Japanese moving to live in the United States frequently develop western diseases typical of US citizens. Even in a country such as Britain, there is a variable difference in the incidence of disease of nutritional origin in different parts of the country: cardiovascular disease is more common in the North-West than in the South-East, and in the West of Scotland than in the East; stomach cancer is particularly common in parts of Wales.

Sir Robert McCarrison (1878–1960), when working in India, was impressed by the differences in physique and disease patterns of different races, which he concluded was caused by their different diets. He proved this in 1926 by taking seven groups each consisting of 20 young rats which he fed on the typical diets of the seven races (Sikhs, Madrassi, etc.). The increase in body weight of the seven groups of rats corresponded to the physique of the seven races, and so did the diseases that the rats developed.

McCarrison lived for seven years as the only medical officer amongst the Hunzas, who inhabit a pocket of the Himalayas. They were notoriously long-lived, of superb physique and endurance. Among the tribe of about 10 000, he saw no case of heart disease, cancer, appendicitis, peptic ulcer, multiple sclerosis or diabetes mellitus. This he attributed to their excellent, almost entirely vegetarian, diet of whole grains, vegetables and fruits.

But the exact opposite of the vegetarian Hunzas were the traditionally carnivorous Eskimos, amongst whom I have lived. They also were virtually free of western disease when living off their traditional diet of seal and fish with sometimes caribou (reindeer) and some berries in summer. Their diet was the highest in fat in the world, but very rich in essential fatty acids.

Lord Boyd Orr, with Gilks, studied in 1931 the physique and health of the Masai and Kikuyu in Kenya. The Masai subsisted largely on the milk, meat and raw blood of their cattle, the Kikuyu mainly on cereals, roots and fruits. Therefore, the Masai had a relatively high intake of protein, fat and calcium, whereas the diet of the Kikuyu was high in carbohydrate and low in calcium. The adult Masai was 13 cm taller and 10.5 kg heavier than the adult Kikuyu, and his strength 50% greater; apart from constipation and rheumatoid arthritis, which were common in the Masai, the Kikuyu had a much higher prevalence of diseases such as dental caries, anaemia, tropical ulcers, pneumonia and bony deformities.

Much work has been done on mineral nutrition, and the prevalence of goitre and its links with iodine deficiency have already been mentioned in Chapter 3. In recent years, selenium has attracted attention. In 1957 Schwartz showed it was an essential nutrient for rats, and it was later found to be an essential component of the enzyme glutathione peroxidase, which destroys lipid peroxides and protects cell membranes against oxidative damage. In some areas of China the soil is poor in selenium, and heart disease results in children (Keshan's disease), but in other areas there is too much and toxicity results. In North America, soils are too high in selenium in parts of Wyoming and the Dakotas, and livestock develop toxicity. Pollution with aluminium, lead, mercury, cadmium and the salts of various other elements also causes disease in man.

Cultural and religious taboos related to food have been studied in relation to disease. There may be feasts, such as excessive consumption of pig-meat in Papua New Guinea, leading to acute necrotic enteritis; or there may be fasts, such as Ramadan (practised by Muslims), which tend to cause a rise in blood uric acid and triacylglycerols. In Ethiopia, there are over 100 fast days in the year, and protein deficiency can occur in vulnerable groups on account of this.   Mahatma Ghandi described the prohibition of killing cows as 'the one concrete belief common to all Hindus'; it once served a useful purpose when the cow was so important in farming, but now the quantities of useless cows in India contribute to malnutrition.

Mormons, who eat meat but do not smoke, and Seventh-day Adventists, most of whom are vegetarians, have less coronary heart disease than others in the US.   In general, vegetarians have fewer western diseases than omnivores in the same locality, but vegans (who will not even eat honey, since it has been touched by a bee) have, on occasion, died of deficiency of vitamin B_{12} before supplements of this isolated from microorganisms became available. Unlike man, true herbivores such as horses have adapted to a plant diet by absorbing the vitamin after synthesis by microorganisms in their intestines.

There is still much work to be done in studying the distribution of disease in relation to diet, and even the study of persons who practise odd fads and fancies in their diets.

Trends in disease patterns
My interest in nutrition as a student arose from noticing that we haven't done much to keep a middle-aged man alive during this century.   Nearly a century and a half ago, when statistics started, the expectation of life of a middle-aged man was much the same as it is now.

Table 5.1 — Comparisons of the changes in expectation of life and causes of death of a man aged 50 years, over the past century and a half.

	1841	1980
Expectation of life (years)	20.0	22.7
Main killing diseases	Tuberculosis, pneumonia	'Western' (cardiovascular, cancer etc.)
Unimportant diseases	Chronic, degenerative or 'western'	Tuberculosis, pneumonia
Anaesthesia, antiseptics, X-rays, hormones, vitamins, antibiotics, modern drugs	No	Yes

In 1841 when statistics were first collected in the UK (Table 5.1), a man aged 50 years could expect to live a further 20 years (i.e. a man of 50 could expect to live to the age of 70).   Today the number of years is only 23 – almost no change. On the other hand, the expectation of life at birth has increased enormously, because many of the infectious diseases, which took such a toll of infants and children, have been abolished. This has occurred partly by better sanitation and partly by better nutrition.

Similar figures apply to the United States, although records there start around 1900. In the UK in 1941, the diseases which were then killing middle-aged men were tuberculosis (TB) and pneumonia, which are unimportant today in this country. The western 'diseases of affluence' were unimportant then: cases of cancer and heart disease were few. The year 1841 was before all the great advances in medicine, before anaesthesia, before the use of antiseptics and almost all the drugs we use today. Despite all these advances we cannot do much more to keep a middle-aged man alive today than in the dark ages — and that is an astounding fact.

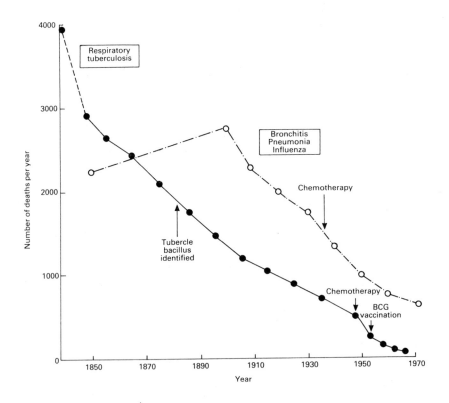

Fig. 5.2 — Trends in death rate in England and Wales due to infections.

The lack of impact of drugs can be illustrated further by the example of TB. Fig. 5.2 shows that in 1841 the deathrate from TB was very high, and yet today it is unimportant in this country. It is of interest that innovations in chemotherapy did not contribute very significantly to this. The decrease in incidence of TB was occurring before the introduction of modern drugs. This was due to better food, nutrition in general, and sanitation. Similarly with pneumonia, the incidence declined before the introduction of chemotherapy. On the other hand, 'diseases of affluence' have been increasing dramatically and nutrition has had a big part to play in this. Fig. 5.3 summarizes some of these changes.

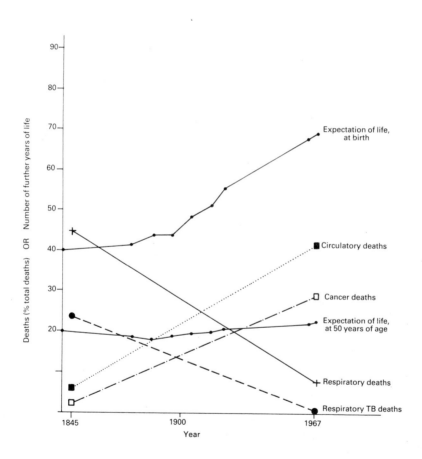

Fig. 5.3 — Trends in expectation of life (males) and causes of death (males aged 50 years).

Disease patterns in various countries

Diseases of affluence are listed in Table 5.2. None of those diseases occurs in Eskimos on their traditional diet. I mention Eskimos because I have worked with them, but similar observations have been made in many parts of the Third World. Diseases such as

Table 5.2 — Western diseases influenced by diet

Circulation	Cancer	Digestive system	Nervous system
Atherosclerosis	Lung	Dental caries	Multiple sclerosis
Coronary heart disease	Breast	Peptic ulcer	Schizophrenia
Hypertension	Colon	Hiatus hernia	Tardive dyskinesia
Cerebro-vascular disease	Rectum	Gall-stones	Migraine
Peripheral vascular disease	Prostate	Appendicitis	
Thrombosis	Stomach	Ulcerative colitis	
Varicose veins		Crohn's disease	
		Diverticulitis	
		Haemorrhoids	
		Cystic fibrosis	
Muscles	*Pregnancy*	*Skin*	*Allergic*
Bones	*Child-birth*		*Endocrine*
Joints			*Metabolic*
			Auto-immune
Osteoporosis	Pre-eclampsia	Acne vulgaris	Obesity
Slipped discs	Breast-pain	Eczema	Asthma
Rheumatoid arthritis	Pre-menstral tension	Psoriasis	Diabetes mellitus
	Anencephaly		Gout
	Spina bifida		Pernicious anaemia
	Down's syndrome		Sjogren's syndrome
			Systemic lupus erythematosus
			Infantile hypercalcaemia

coronary heart disease (see Chapter 7) and cancer are, on the whole, diseases of developed countries. The great Arctic explorer, Stefansson, whom I knew well, marshalled evidence in his last book 'Cancer: disease of civilisation?' that, in Third World countries, except for two forms of cancer, namely aflatoxin-induced primary cancer of the liver and Burkitt's lymphoma, cancer was a rare disease until recently. He pointed out that malignant disease was totally unknown among traditional Eskimos. Indeed, the first case among them was described as late as 1952. Unfortunately, it is now becoming quite common. Since 1950 almost all Eskimos have been colonized by Americans, eat American-style diets and get American disease patterns.

Multiple sclerosis is a horrible disease, very common in developed countries. It is almost unknown in Africa and China, and extremely rare in Japan. On the whole, all 'diseases of affluence' are rare in Japan (although they are now starting to increase), except two. The Japanese in Japan frequently get cancer of the stomach but not of other organs. They also get high blood pressure, leading to high prevalence of strokes. We believe (it is not proved) that these two conditions are associated with their diets being very high in salt.

UNDERNUTRITION

Table 5.3 — Third World diseases influenced by diet

Children	Adults
Kwashiorkor	Starvation
Marasmus	Xerophthalmia
Xerophthalmia	Cataract
(blindness)	Anaemia
Rickets	Goitre and Cretinism
Scurvy	Cancer of the liver

Protein energy malnutrition

In the Third World the pattern of disease is very different from that in the industrialized world (Table 5.3) and, in children, kwashiorkor and marasmus dominate. These are collectively called protein-energy malnutrition and represent the extreme manifestations of this deficiency. These illnesses are both regrettably common, but are very different in appearance. Kwashiorkor occurs mainly in children between the ages of two and five years, whereas marasmus is a condition of infants. Marasmus is pure starvation and the infant is wasted.

Kwashiorkor is common in West Africa and the name is derived from the Ghanian (Ga) word meaning 'the disease which kills the first-born infant when the second infant comes along'. It is normal practice in that part of the world for a mother to nurse her baby even into the second year of life, until she becomes pregnant again. The child is often late-weaned onto a starchy gruel. If this is derived from manioc (also called cassava — a tuber) or plantain (a crop similar to banana) then the protein content of the diet will be very low. Infants suffering from protein-energy malnutrition are deprived of protein often for two reasons. First, the energy intake is lower than requirements, which means that protein in the diet is used to provide energy and not used for its primary purpose of growth and maintenance, and secondly the weaning food is low in protein.

Vitamin A deficiency

Supplementation of the diet with dried skimmed milk is one way of treating kwashiorkor, although care must be taken that xerophthalmia is not precipitated and that the child being treated is not lactose intolerant (see Chapter 4). Xerophthalmia is a deficiency disease of retinol (vitamin A), very prevalent in certain parts of the world, and largely affecting children. The cornea of the eye (which is the clear, front part of the eyeball) becomes dry, shrivelled and opaque and then cracks, leading to infection and, if untreated, blindness. It can be treated by corneal grafts, but this needs the supply of corneas from the deceased, which are not easily obtained, especially from those of the Hindu faith. The problem is being tackled well in parts of India by encouraging the growing of green vegetables (containing β-carotene), although deficiency is still prevalent in many parts of Africa. In Africa it is especially common where there is no red palm oil in the diet. Red palm oil is a very good source of β-carotene which the body can convert to vitamin A.

Fish are a very good source of the vitamin, particularly fish livers. In Uganda there is an area called the 'River of the blind', which is a horrible place, where the children who are going blind lead around adults who are blind. There are fish in the river, but there is a taboo on eating them!

In India there are excellent medical eye camps. An ophthalmologist, a nurse and a dietitian travel to the villages and set up a camp. People come from far and wide to bring the infants suffering from malnutrition, who are given injections with sufficient vitamin A to last six months. More cannot be given, as vitamin A is toxic in excess. Of course, injections can only be considered a temporary measure; the best course would be to educate people to grow and eat green leafy vegetables so that there is plenty of β-carotene in the diet.

Blindness caused by malnutrition also occurs in adults. In particular, cataract (opacity of the lens of the eye) can be a serious problem, particularly in India. The causes of this condition are not understood, but it is probably caused by deficiency of nutritional antioxidants, vitamin E, β-carotene, ascorbic acid and selenium. Unfortunately, there are charlatans called 'coushers' in India, who make a lot of money out of this condition. These 'coushers' use a thorn or needle to displace the opaque lens, so that the patient is able to see. The quack takes his fee and moves on. In a short time the patient becomes permanently blinded in both eyes. This happens because infection sets in in the eye 'operated' on, and lens protein gets broken down. Lens protein is not a protein which the body is accustomed to meet and, therefore, antibodies are produced against it, which act against the lens protein of the other eye, which is then destroyed, leading to complete blindness.

ESSENTIAL FATTY ACIDS (EFA)

I wish to discuss essential fatty acids because I believe that many of our western diseases of affluence are mainly caused by a relative deficiency of EFA, which means a low ratio in the body of EFA to long-chain saturated fatty acids and isomers of EFA (*trans* fatty acids), both of which are antagonistic to the function of EFA. Of course, excess sugar in the diet is converted in the body to long-chain saturated fatty acids, so sugar, too, is implicated. As an illustration of the role of EFA in disease conditions, I start with a disease which arose unexpectedly in the UK not long ago.

In 1952, quite suddenly, it was found that infants were being severely affected by too much calcium, and some infants died of this. Two government committees, one by the Ministry of Health and the other by the Medical Research Council, were set up; I was a member of them both. We looked very carefully into what was happening. All affected children were being fed cow's milk preparations. The food manufacturers were adding high amounts of vitamin D, which were leading to hypercalcaemia. We were able to obtain from mothers information on the amounts of artificial milk that had been fed to the infant each day. Hypercalcaemia could arise with as little as 600 IU of vitamin D daily, which is not a toxic dose. Both committees concluded that this condition was caused by increased susceptibility of the infants to vitamin D, rather than the infants being given an excessive amount.

I was very interested in this because there were three signs in infantile hypercalcaemia which do not arise with normal vitamin D toxicity. One was brain damage: certain of the infants became imbeciles, and by using X-rays it was shown that this was not due to calcium deposition, as would be expected as a consequence of vitamin D toxicity if it had affected the brain. Other signs were a raised plasma cholesterol level and hypertension. (A distinguished paediatrician stated that the latter was caused by atherosclerosis.)

I suspected that the answer might lie with essential fatty acid (EFA) deficiency, as cow's milk is an exceedingly poor source of EFA and human milk an excellent source. So we did a simple experiment. Rats deficient in EFA and pair-fed control rats were given a non-toxic dose of vitamin D and in two weeks the rats deficient in EFA were dead, owing to calcification of the kidneys. Thus, we showed that in EFA deficiency there was increased susceptibility to vitamin D toxicity. It was interesting that the hypercalcaemia in infants had occurred in the UK and Scandinavia, but not in the USA. In fact, there was a difference in the formulations of formula milks in these countries. Infant formulas were based on dried cow's milk in the UK and Scandinavia at the time, and during processing, dried cow's milk loses what little EFA it contains; while in the USA evaporated milks were used, which still retained their small amount of EFA.

Metabolism of essential fatty acids

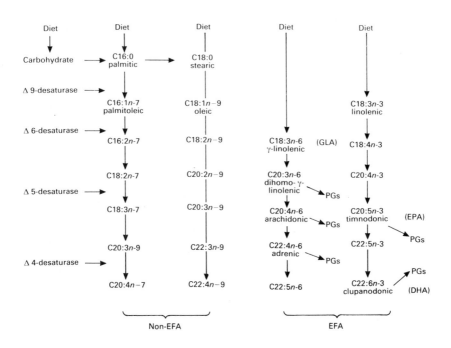

Fig. 5.4 — Metabolism of the various classes of dietary fatty acids. (EFA, essential fatty acid; EPA, eicosapentaenoic acid; DHA, docosahexaenoic acid; GLA, gamma linolenic acid; PG, prostanoids.)

Fig. 5.4 shows the pathways of essential fatty acid metabolism in the body. At the top left-hand side of Fig. 5.4 it shows two dietary saturated fatty acids, palmitic and stearic (C16 and C18). The body can desaturate and elongate stearic acid to give first oleic acid (the commonest fatty acid in both animals and plants) and then elongate it to a fatty acid with 20 carbons and 3 double bonds, **eicosatrienoic**; but this latter conversion only occurs in the body if it is deficient in EFA.

On the right-hand side of Figure 5.4, two different families of EFA, the linoleic and the linolenic, are illustrated: linoleic (18 carbons) with 2 double bonds and linolenic (18 carbons) with 3 double bonds. These are denoted omega-6 and omega-3 unsaturated fatty acids, respectively, (or more correctly, n-6 and n-3). The designation 'omega'-6 or -3 indicates where the first double bond comes, counting from the methyl end of the fatty acid chain. Each of these fatty acids can be desaturated and elongated in the body, to give rise to conversions from linoleic acid to arachidonic acid (probably the most important EFA) and from linolenic acid to timnodonic (C20 with 5 double bonds) and to clupanodonic (C22 with 6 double bonds), which are often considered as the 'marine fatty acids' as they are found in high quantities in fish oils; they are more correctly described as **eicosapentaenoic** (EPA) and **docosahexaenoic** (DHA), respectively.

The conversion of linoleic acid (C18:2n-6) to arachidonic (C20:4n-6) is done by two enzymes, a Δ-6 desaturase, which converts linoleic to γ-linolenic (C18:3n-6), and a Δ-5 desaturase which converts dihomo-γ-linolenic (C20:3n-6) to arachidonic. These enzymes, particularly the first, are easily inhibited by, for instance, aging, diabetes, alcohol, high cholesterol, deficiency of zinc or of vitamins B_6 or C, viruses, glucocorticoids etc. This inhibition can be remedied by administering γ-linolenic acid (GLA) itself, and Evening Primrose oil is an excellent source. A large number of clinical trials with this in various diseases have now been conducted, and are admirably reviewed in a very recent book: *Omega-6 Essential Fatty Acids* (1990) D. F. Horrobin, (ed.) A. R. Liss, New York.

The reason that fish oils are largely derived from linolenic acid is that, whereas linoleic acid is mainly found in seeds, linolenic acid is the predominant fatty acid in leaves (grass, for instance, has 65 % of its fatty acids as linolenic). In the marine environment, the phytoplankton are the botanic equivalent to leaves, and these occupy the head of the long marine food chain. Phytoplankton are eaten by small fish, which elongate and desaturate the linolenic acid. Small fish are eaten by larger fishes etc. and by seals. The outcome is that the fat of marine fish and animals contains a high proportion of long-chain fatty acids with a large number of unsaturated bonds (EPA and DHA). These are now being produced as fish oil supplements for the prevention and treatment of certain medical conditions, which will be alluded to below.

The functions of EFA
The functions of EFA are threefold (Table 5.4). By far the most important function is in the structure of cell membranes.

Cell membranes
All membranes of the cells of animals, whether they be plasma, mitochondrial or other, are formed by a double row of phospholipids, some protein and free cholesterol.

Table 5.4 — Functions of essential fatty acids

- *Phospholipids of cellular membranes*

    — Plasma, mitochondrial, nuclear, lysosomal,
    red blood cell, etc.

- *Transport and oxidation of cholesterol*

    — Transport to cells in LDL.
    — Transport from cells as cholesterol linoleate in HDL.
    — Oxidation in liver to bile acids.

- *Formation of prostanoids*

    — Prostaglandins, thromboxanes,
    prostacyclins, leukotrienes.

HDL, high density lipoproteins; LDL, low density lipoproteins.

Invariably, one of the two fatty acids in the phospholipid molecule is an EFA. A characteristic feature of the presence of a double bond in an EFA is the 'kink' or bend which it imparts to the chain; so arachidonic acid with its 4 double bonds is like a horseshoe, curled right round. It is believed that the cholesterol in cell membranes is fitted into the curves of the EFA. We can explain almost all of the conditions that arise from deficiency of EFA in terms of defects in cellular membranes. Where cellular membranes are being formed, if there is an excess of saturated or monounsaturated fatty acids — the type that the body can make from carbohydrate — then that gets incorporated, leading to faulty membranes being formed, which are very susceptible to a variety of insults.

Lipid transport
The transport of lipids in the blood is accomplished by the formation of lipoproteins. Low density **lipoproteins** (LDL) transport EFA to cells, and high density lipoproteins (HDL) remove excess cholesterol from the tissues to the liver where it can be converted into bile acids and excreted. Further aspects of lipid transport are dealt with in Chapter 7.

Prostaglandins and related substances
Prostanoids, including prostaglandins, can only be formed from essential fatty acids. When this was first discovered the belief was then held by some people that the function of EFA was solely to produce prostaglandins. However, we know now that this is not so, from some very interesting research which has been carried out by Unilever in Holland on a fatty acid called columbinic acid (Fig. 5.5), which was isolated from columbine seeds.

COLUMBINIC ACID

$$\overset{cis}{}\qquad\overset{cis}{}\qquad\overset{trans}{}$$

$$CH_3 - (CH_2)_4 - CH{=}CH - CH_2 - \ CH{=}CH - (CH_2)_2 - CH{=}CH - (CH_2)_3 - COOH$$

LINOLEIC ACID

$$\overset{cis}{}\qquad\overset{cis}{}$$

$$CH_3 - (CH_2)_4 - CH{=}CH - CH_2 - CH{=}CH - (CH_2)_7 - COOH$$

Fig. 5.5 — Comparison of the structures of columbinic acid and linoleic acid.

This fatty acid has a similar structure to linoleic acid (see Fig. 5.5), with 18 carbons and 2 double bonds in the same place, but it has an extra (3rd) double bond in the *trans* configuration. If columbinic acid is given to a rats on a fat-free diet, it prevents all the signs of EFA deficiency except kidney lesions. It is now known that columbinic acid cannot be converted into prostanoids (it is not a substrate for cyclo-oxygenase — an enzyme involved in prostanoid formation). This is an excellent demonstration that the major functions of EFA are not associated with the production of prostanoids.

In Fig. 5.6 linoleic acid is shown with its conversion to arachidonic acid, which then goes to form prostaglandins which cause blood platelets to disaggregate (not to stick together). Also included in Fig. 5.6 is an important compound called prostacyclin, which is also very powerful in disaggregating blood platelets. However, **thromboxane (TXA$_2$)** is also produced in the metabolic pathway from arachidonic acid and this makes platelets aggregate (stick together), causing blood clotting or thrombosis. An interesting point is that if you switch from a diet which is rich in linoleic acid or arachidonic acid (and therefore making thromboxane TXA$_2$, which makes platelets aggregate — note that lean meat is a good source of arachidonic acid), to a diet rich in fish oils then you get a prostaglandin which disaggregates platelets, a prostacyclin which also disaggregates platelets, and, in addition, a thromboxane that has no effect on platelets. So the biologically active metabolic products from dietary fish oils prevent thrombosis in comparison with dietary linoleic or arachidonic acids.

Coronary heart disease and EFA
As explained in Chapter 7, most coronary heart disease (CHD) is preceded by atherosclerosis, but it is a thrombosis which will normally precipitate a heart attack. Although in many western countries, such as Britain, it is common to find that atherosclerosis and thrombosis are prevalent in the same community, these conditions are not inextricably linked, as has been shown by epidemiological observation. Fig. 5.7 shows the classes of fatty acids which are antagonistic to EFA and the effects of the

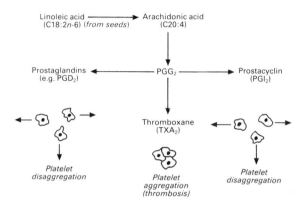

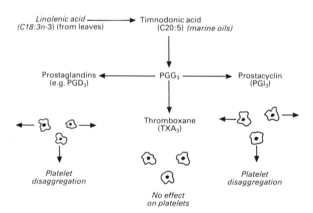

Fig. 5.6 — Essential fatty acids and the formation of prostanoids. (EPA, eicosapentaenoic acid; PG, prostaglandin.)

various fatty acid classes on platelet aggregation (involved in thrombosis) and changes in blood cholesterol level (involved in development of atherosclerosis).

There are certain countries in the world such as Jamaica, Cuba and the Cook Islands, where atherosclerosis is very prevalent, but thrombosis is rare. This results from high intakes of coconut oil containing two saturated fatty acids, lauric and myristic acids (C12 and C14), which produce atherosclerosis but do not lead to thrombosis.

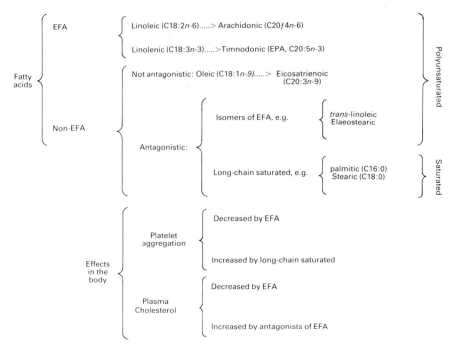

Fig. 5.7 — Interrelationships of essential fatty acids (EFA) and non-essential fatty acids (non-EFA), and their effects in the body. (EPA, eicosapentaenoic acid.)

Analysis of human adipose tissue for linoleic acid can be a useful indicator of diet. As linoleic acid cannot be made in the body, that in the adipose tissue can only come from the diet, and therefore can be used as an indication of the dietary linoleic acid. Fig. 5.8 shows the linoleic acid content of human adipose tissue, which has been analysed from tissue biopsies. Data for the USA are on the upper plots in Fig. 5.8. The filled circles are published mean values for the amount of linoleic acid in adipose tissue since 1956.

From Fig. 5.8, it is clear that the contribution of linoleic acid in adipose tissue in the USA remained at about 10% of the total fatty acids until 1968, since when the proportion of linoleic acid has increased dramatically. Since that time, deaths from CHD have also dropped dramatically by over 30% in the USA. The crosses in Fig. 5.8 represent the reciprocal of the death rate due to coronary heart disease (so the drop in deaths is shown by the rise in the reciprocal plot in Fig. 5.8). Thus the two sets of information fit beautifully.

On the lower plot of Fig. 5.8 are the equivalent data for the UK. Values for linoleic acid start slightly lower and they are only now beginning to rise slightly. Deaths from CHD (not shown) in the UK have remained at a constant high level and are only just now starting to fall. So that is a good indication that dietary linoleic acid is important in CHD.

Also plotted in Fig. 5.8 are the author's adipose tissue, linoleic acid levels, while on and Eskimo diet, described in the next section.

Other Diseases and EFA
Table 5.5 shows that the incidence of different types of cancer varies considerably from one country to another. In Africa, deaths from all forms of cancer are very low

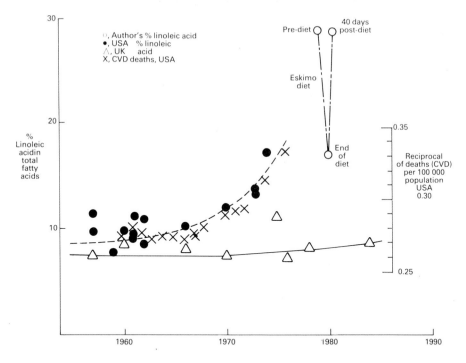

Fig. 5.8 — Changes over some years in linoleic acid content of human adipose tissue in the USA compared with the UK, and changes in author's tissue when on Eskimo diet (fish, seal and water).

compared with western countries, except for primary liver cancer caused by aflatoxin from groundnuts. Of particular note is how rare cancer is in Japan, except for cancer of the stomach, where it is exceedingly high (as already mentioned).

(Incidentally, it is of great interest that there is very little cancer of the lung in Japan, although the prevalence of smoking in Japan is higher than in any other country of the world, with the possible exception of the Eskimos today. That is very interesting and points to the involvement of a nutritional factor, such as a relatively high dietary content of EFA. Although I am strongly opposed to smoking, smoking alone is not the whole story in the development of lung cancer.)

Table 5.5 — Incidence of different types of cancer worldwide
(annual rate per 100 000 males aged 35–64)

Country		Stomach	Colon	Lung	Liver (Primary)	Breast (women)
Africa	(Mozambique)	5	5	0	165	10
America	(NY State)	17	27	65	0	103
Asia	(Japan)	158	5	23	0	33
Europe	(Iceland)	102	9	28	0	84
"	(Scotland)	43	28	154	0	111
"	(England — SE)	31	16	128	0	103

Source: Doll, 1969.

Eskimos are an extremely interesting human group in that, living on their traditional diet, the highest in the world in fat, but very rich in EFA, they had none of our western diseases. Table 5.6 compares the traditional diet of the Eskimo with the diets of some other human groups. I have made a special study of this group. On my return from the last study I decided to live on an 'Eskimo diet' for 100 days. This comprised only fish, seal (muscle, liver and blubber) and water.

Table 5.6 — Dietary fat in some typical adult male diets

Dietary fat	British Usual	British Vegetarian	Poor Indian	Japanese farmer	Traditional Eskimo
Total dietary fat	High	Low	Low	Very low	Very high
g/day	117	—	44	30	200
% energy	42	—	15	11	60
Major EFA	C18:2n-6	C18:3n-3 C18:2n-6	C18:2n-6	C18:3n-3 C20:5n-3 C22:6n-3	C20:5n-3 C22:6n-3
Saturated fat	High	Low	Very low	Very low	High
g/day	53		10	7	49
Trans fatty acids	High	Variable	Negligible	Negligible	Zero
P/S ratio	Very low 0.2	High	Very high 1.0	Very high 1.4	Very high 1.0

P/S ratio, (polyunsaturates/saturates), $\dfrac{\text{EFA}}{\text{saturated} + trans \text{ FA}}$; EFA, essential fatty acids.

Changes in dietary fat intake can be monitored by the changes in incorporation of fatty acids into compounds such as phospholipids, which are part of the membrane structure of cells (see above). Fig. 5.9 shows the content of the three main fatty acids, linoleic, arachidonic and eicosapentaenoic (EPA) (in that order), in platelet phospholipids before and after the 100-day Eskimo diet. Consider the phospholipid, phosphatidylethanolamine. It can be seen that the arachidonic acid content is very high before the diet, and drops down very dramatically after; EPA rose very dramatically on the Eskimo diet. Fig. 5.8 shows the changes in linoleic acid in my adipose tissue, the Eskimo diet being very low in this fatty acid.

One result of the changes in platelet phospholipids was the very great alteration in my bleeding time (Fig. 5.10). (Bleeding time is measured by making a small slit in the skin and noting the time that is required for the bleeding to stop). Normal bleeding time is 3 - 4 minutes, but in Greenland Eskimos it is about 10 minutes. During my diet the bleeding time went up to more than 50 minutes, which caused spontaneous haemorrhages, including nose bleeds. Dramatic alterations in thrombotic activity can, therefore, be produced by changing the EFA in the diet.

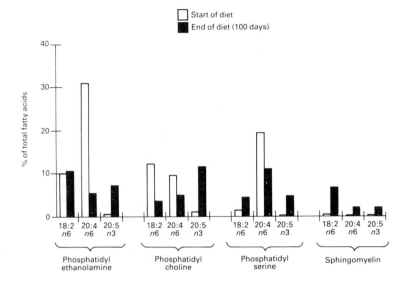

Fig. 5.9 — Changes in fatty acid content (linoleic, arachidonic and eicosapentaenoic acids) of platelet phospholipids of author after 100 days on an Eskimo diet.

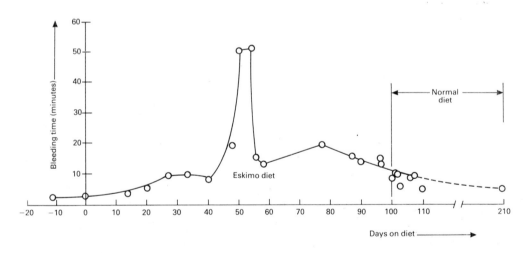

Fig. 5.10 — Changes in the bleeding time of author during 100 days on an Eskimo diet.

CLINICAL SIGNS OF MALNUTRITION AND THE IMPORTANCE OF CORRECT DIAGNOSIS

Vitamin A Deficiency

Plate 5.1 shows the skin of a forearm with **follicular hyperkeratosis**, sometimes called 'nutmeg-grater' skin. The skin is rough, and this sign occurs early in vitamin A deficiency, although it is of no great diagnostic significance, unlike the effects of

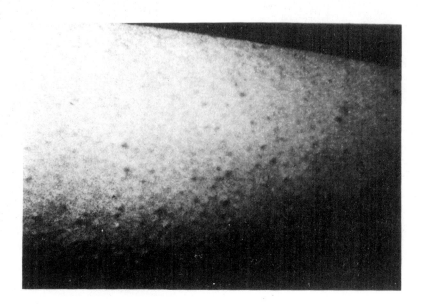

Plate 5.1 — Hyperkeratosis ('nutmeg-grater' skin): an early sign of vitamin A deficiency.

protracted vitamin A deficiency, which lead to xerophthalmia which has already been mentioned. The first observable result of deficiency of retinol is impaired vision in the dark (see Chapter 3). Deficiency of retinol occurs in Central America (e.g. Guatemala), throughout about half of Africa, where there is no red palm oil, in the Middle East and across India to the Far East (e.g. Malaysia).

Vitamin D Deficiency
Vitamin D deficiency causes rickets in children and osteomalacia in adults. Rickets first became prevalent in Britain around 1620, perhaps because the Reformation caused less fish to be eaten.   In rickets, the growing bones are weak from deficiency of calcium, which is absorbed from the intestine with the aid of vitamin D. The weak bones bend easily.   The disease can occur in sunny climates if children are wrapped in clothes so that sunlight does not form vitamin D in the skin. Cases have been appearing in this country in recent years among Asian immigrants.

Thiamin Deficiency
Plate 5.2 shows a case of beri-beri, although you might mistakenly think that the woman in Plate 5.2(a) was very obese.   Beri-beri manifests in two forms: **dry beri-beri**, which is accompanied by alteration of the nervous system, sometimes leading to inability to walk; and **wet beri-beri** (which is the form shown in Plate 5.2), in which there is

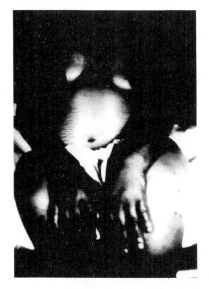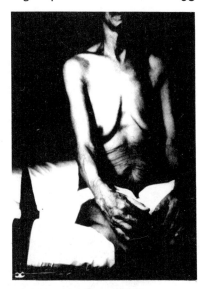

Plate 5.2 — (a) A woman with wet beri-beri (severe deficiency of thiamin). (b) The same woman showing a rapid reponse to thiamin treatment.

retention of fluid. Plate 5.2(a) does not show obesity: such a case will respond rapidly to thiamin treatment, as is shown in Plate 5.2(b). Beri-beri is found among rice-eating peoples (more than half the world's population): it used to be very prevalent in the Far East associated with diets high in polished rice.

There is also a condition of acute thiamin deficiency called Wernicke's encephalopathy, which has severe effects on mental function. Fortunately it is not common, but I remember in 1940 seeing one patient who was completely mad. We gave her intravenous thiamin (which had been first synthesized four years earlier) and within a day she was walking out of hospital. It is one of the most dramatic results of food and nutritional science that can be observed. The patient is brought into hospital raving mad and, after intravenous thiamin is administered, the condition is cured — quickly and completely reversed. However, until about 1940 Wernicke's encephalopathy was invariably fatal in a matter of hours.

Riboflavin deficiency
This condition is quite prevalent in certain parts of the world. Riboflavin is one of the B vitamins, and in 1938 deficiency was characterized in man. Blood vessels grow across the front of the eye (cornea), but these clinical manifestations are not as important as the lesions which occur at muco-cutaneous junctions (areas where mucous membranes and skin join), such as eyelids, ears, base of the nose, lips and around the genital region (Plate 5.3). Often those deficient in riboflavin show photophobia, closing the eyes, and also show the characteristic change in the tongue, which is purple and swollen.

Nicotinic acid (niacin) deficiency
Nicotinic acid deficiency results in **pellagra,** a condition in which a severe skin rash

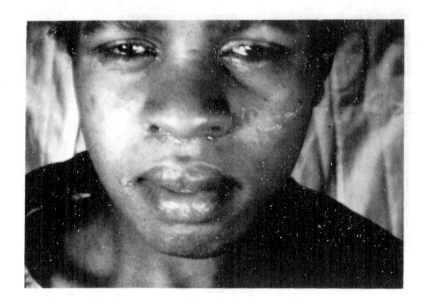

Plate 5.3 — Riboflavin deficiency shows in lesions at mucocutaneous junctions (seen here at eyelids, base of nose and lips).

(dermatitis) occurs, which is sharply limited to areas exposed to sun (Plate 5.4). The tongue of the pellagrin is bright red and atrophied and is quite different from the tongue in riboflavin deficiency, which is purple and swollen. Pellagra was a very important deficiency disease in the Southern USA until the 1940s, and is still found in maize-eating areas of Africa, India and Italy, Central America and Mexico. It is sometimes called the 3 Ds — causing dermatitis, dementia, and diarrhoea (inflammation of the gut involves the entire gut from the tongue to the anus). The dementia is particularly important.

Some years ago I had sent to me a pellagrin who had been put into a mental hospital. She was a farmer's wife who was diagnosed as being insane and she happened to sit out in the sun and got a dermatitis. The consultant dermatologist sent her to me and I diagnosed her as a pellagrin. With treatment with nicotinic acid she was completely cured and went back to the farm.   In the past, other people diagnosed as insane have been confined to mental hospitals in this country, when, in fact, they were deficient in a nutrient.   Some of them have not been fortunate enough to sit in the sun and get skin rashes. So we have to be very careful in diagnosis.

Vitamin C Deficiency
One of the characteristic features of scurvy is the bleeding of gums around the teeth. It occurs in the UK among elderly people, but is also called 'batchelor's scurvy' as it often occurs in people who eat food from tins and forgo eating fresh fruit and vegetables. However, bleeding gums are only a sign of scurvy and then only if the person has teeth.

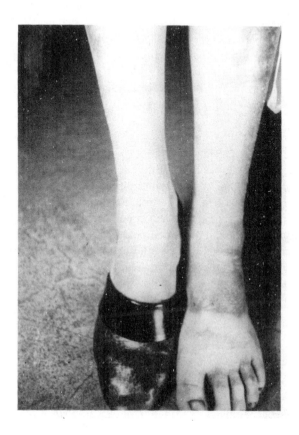

Plate 5.4 — Nicotinic acid deficiency causes pellagra, which is characterized by a skin rash sharply limited to areas exposed to the sun.

Many people over the age of 40 in the UK are edentulous; therefore, if they get scurvy they will not have bleeding gums. Several years ago an important person in charge of nutrition at the Ministry of Health used a metal probe for pressing on gums to test whether they would bleed. He found that in people over the age of 40 he got virtually no bleeding and was surprised that the results indicated that scurvy decreased after middle-age. However, he had failed to note those people in the survey who were edentulous.

There is one sign in scurvy which is pathognomonic, which means it occurs in scurvy and no other clinical disorder. The sign is the presence of tiny pinpoint haemorrhages around the hair follicles. Neverthess, care has to be taken during examination to arrive at the correct diagnosis even in this case, as will be seen in the following example, which shows how easily misinterpreted clinical signs can be.

Just after the 1939–1945 war I went with experts from the other three Allies, USSR,

USA and France, to assess the nutritional situation in Germany. The Germans tried to make as much of their alleged nutritional deficiencies as possible, as they knew that the outcome of our investigations would be to fix ration scales and they wanted then to be as high as possible. In Dusseldorf an American colleague called me across to look at a man who was described as having scurvy. He had pinpoint haemorrhages, but they were not around hair follicles, but between them. It was clear that he could not have scurvy. I asked the patient how long it was since he last had a bath and he replied that he had never had a bath until the previous evening. He had been dragged out of a gutter, washed and brushed up, given a clean pair of pyjamas and labelled 'scurvy'. In fact, he had vagabond's disease — lice bites. Lice produce pinpoint haemorrhages, but they avoid the hairs and bite nice bits of naked skin between the hairs!

CONCLUSION

So, if you have a rough skin or cracks at the corners of your mouth or gums that bleed when you brush them, or (and I am sure not) pin point haemorrhages between hairs, do not assume you are malnourished. Malnutrition is a term encompassing both under- and over-nutrition, both of which conditions are of concern to the food and nutrition scientist. Diet is a key feature in maintaining good health. There are many healthy long-lived people who are strict vegetarians (vegans) and there are people who are also mainly free from western disease of affluence (such as traditional Eskimos and the Masai) who are carnivores. By the correlation of diets and disease in different groups of peoples, the food and nutritional sciences are greatly helping medicine.

REFERENCES

Armstrong, B. K. and Doll, R. (1975) Environmental factors and cancer incidence and mortality in different countries with special reference to dietary practices. *International Journal of Cancer*. **15**, 617–631.

Doll, R. (1969) The geographical distribution of cancer. *British Journal of Cancer*. **23**, 1–8.

Katan, M. B. and Beynen, A. C. (1981) Linoleic acid consumption and coronary heart disease in the USA and UK. *Lancet, ii*, 371.

Lancet Editorial (1983). Eskimo diets and diseases. *Lancet* i, 1139-1141.

McCarrison, R. (1953) *The work of Sir Robert McCarrison* (Sinclair, H. M., ed.) Faber and Faber, London.

Orr, J. B. and Gilks, J. L. (1931) Studies in nutrition. The physique and health of two African tribes. *Medical Research Council Special Report Series, 155*.

Sinclair, H. M. (1953) The diet of Canadian Indians and Eskimos. *Proceedings of the Nutrition Society* **12**, 69–82.

Sinclair, H. M. (1982) Essential fatty acids (vitamin F). In: Barker, B. M. and Bender, D. A. (eds) *Vitamins in Medicine* Heinemann, London.

Sinclair, H. M. (1987) Food fats good and bad. *British Journal of Clinical Practice*. **41**, 1033–1036.

Stefansson, V. (1960) *Cancer: disease of civilisation?* Hill and Wang, New York.

6

Obesity and its implications for health

Michael Gurr

Introduction

'Obesity' or 'overweight' is today regarded as a serious health problem in the UK at a time when our television screens attest to the fact that many people in the world are starving. We get messages about obesity from the television, women's magazines and newspapers. Health committees tell of its importance and national dietary guidelines always include maintenance of an appropriate body weight as a primary goal (Chapter 1). In addition, many people are undoubtedly trying to lose weight for reasons that have little to do with health. In this chapter the following questions are discussed:

What is obesity ?
How can we measure it ?
How prevalent is it ?
Why is it important for health ?
How do we become obese ?

A major part of the chapter will then be devoted to the question:

How can we lose excess weight ?

This will include a discussion of a range of weight-reduction techniques, the dangers and difficulties associated with weight reduction and the types of foods and diets available for 'slimming'.

WHAT IS OBESITY?

The body is composed of lean and fat tissues. The fat (**adipose**) tissues act as a long-term store of energy to be used as a reserve fuel during starvation and also serve as a means of protecting or insulating the body and the internal organs. Normally, the adipose tissue makes up about a quarter of the body weight in men and a third of the body weight in women. When the adipose tissue weight is considerably more than this we have the condition known as 'obesity' or 'overweight'. There seems to be no 'official' definition of these terms, but as a rough guide we could regard overweight as being above the ideal range of body weight and obesity as the more severe condition in which body weight is more than 20% above the upper end of the acceptable range of weights.

How, then, do we define what is 'ideal'? Clearly, a person can have a large 'frame size' (i.e. very tall, large bone mass, high lean body mass) and not be obese. Thus, it is customary to relate fat mass or total weight to height in order to assess overweight. Ideal weight has come to be associated with a fat mass that carries minimal health risks. The generally accepted assessment of ideal weight comes from life expectancy figures generated by life assurance companies, i.e. a set of weights-for-height that are consistent with the longest life expectancy. Most people studying obesity have used the height–weight tables of the Metropolitan Life Insurance Co. of New York. From these we can construct graphs relating weight to height and can assess whether we are in the ideal range, overweight or underweight for any given height (see Fig. 6.1). In order to express the degree of overweight numerically and compare the body mass of different individuals or populations, various indices have been developed. The most commonly used today is the **Quetelet Index** or '**Body Mass Index**' (BMI).

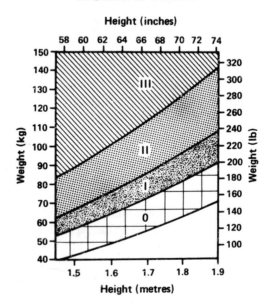

Fig. 6.1 — Degrees of obesity (0, underweight; I, normal; II, overweight; III, obese). Source: Garrow, 1978. Reproduced with permission from Elsevier Science Publishers.

How do we measure obesity?
Table 6.1 shows various indices of overweight which have been used in the past, together with the Body Mass Index (BMI, W/h^2) which, for many purposes, is good enough. It has the merit of being simple to derive with the simplest of equipment. Recommended normal range of BMI is 20 – 25 for men and women.

Table 6.1 — Various indices of overweight

- Percentage above 'ideal' weight
    Overweight if percentage >10%

- Ponderal Index $= \dfrac{\text{height in inches}}{\sqrt[3]{\text{weight in lbs}}}$

    Overweight if index <12

- Fat fold thickness
    Overweight if thickness > 2.5 cm   at top of scapula (men)
                                                            at top mid-triceps (women)

- Quetelet Index or Body Mass Index (BMI)

    BMI $= W/h^2$ where W = weight in kg
                                                h = height in m

Underweight	BMI < 20
Normal	BMI 20–25
Overweight	BMI 25–30
Obese	BMI >30

To be more 'scientific' or accurate we may wish to measure the adipose tissue itself, since this is what actually governs the degree of overweight. The simplest way to do this is by measuring the '**skinfold thickness**' with skinfold callipers (see Plate 2.3). This relies on the fact that much human adipose tissue lies under the skin (subcutaneous adipose tissue) and by pinching a fold of skin we can get some measure of the degree of adiposity. A problem is that adipose tissue is not evenly distributed — some people have more round their thighs, others on their abdomen, etc. Several skinfold measurements are usually made in different anatomical sites and an average taken. Another problem is that fat around the internal organs (e.g. gut, kidneys) is not taken into account. The method has the advantage that it requires only simple, inexpensive apparatus and can be in used in 'field surveys' (e.g. in assessing the incidence of overweight in schoolchildren). Whichever 'simple method' is used, it is generally calibrated against one of the more rigorous scientific methods, such as those measuring density, body water or body radiopotassium.

Data on body measurements on groups of lean and obese subjects in Cambridge, which the author and his colleagues carried out a few years ago give some idea of the range of weights-for-height that can exist in a normal British population (Table 6.2). As implied above, subcutaneous adipose tissue may be distributed differently in different people. People are generally characterized as having an '**android**' or upper body distribution, charactersitic of, but not exclusive to males, or a '**gynoid**' or lower body distribution, characteristic of but not exclusive to, females. Because a large part of the excess adipose tissue in 'upper body obesity' accumulates around the abdomen and in 'lower body obesity' around the thighs, it has become usual to characterize individuals according to the ratio of waist circumference to hip circumference. This is now regarded as an important measurement because of the established metabolic differences between upper and lower body obesity, as described later.

Table 6.2 — Range of BMIs for various groups of adults in Cambridge

Group	Sex	No. in group	Mean weight (kg)	Fat (kg)	W/h^2 (kg/m^2)
Obese	M	19	118± 31	40.4± 16.6	37.4± 7.8
	F	75	93 ± 19	41.0± 8.8	36.0± 7.6
Lean	M	11	69 ± 11	16.2± 6.3	23.1± 2.8
	F	37	59 ± 7	18.6± 5	22.3± 2

± Standard error of mean.
Body Mass Index (BMI) = W/h^2
Source: Gurr et al., 1982.

What is the prevalence of obesity in the UK population?
Surprisingly, very few comprehensive surveys have been carried out on the prevalence of obesity in the UK. However, recent surveys suggest that a very substantial proportion of the UK adult population weighs in excess of the acceptable weight ranges. The prevalence of overweight increases from 15% in 16–19-year-olds to 54% in men and 50% in women aged 60–65 years of age (Table 6.3). If all adults are considered, then 39% of men and 32% of women are overweight (BMI greater than 25). About 14% of the population is thought to have a BMI greater than 27.5, which requires immediate action if it is not to develop into severe obesity. About 6% of men and 8% of women are classified as obese, which constitutes a severe health risk. The average weight-for-height of the population is continuing to rise and this suggests that the population is continuing to become overweight.

The environmental factors accounting for this weight increase are many, including a decline in physical activity and change in dietary patterns. Diets rich in fat and simple sugars and with little dietary fibre are thought to be conducive to weight gain.

Why is obesity thought to be important?
Risks associated with excess weight are not confined only to those who are substantially obese: a progressive increase in morbidity and mortality is apparent with even small increases in weights above the acceptable range. Table 6.4 shows diseases for which obesity imposes an increased risk. Surgical operations are more hazardous because, among other things, the sheer mass of adipose tissue can obscure the internal organs.

Obesity is related to high blood pressure both on an individual and a population basis.

Table 6.3 — Prevalence of obesity in the UK

| | BMI | Percentage of age group | | | | |
		16–19 yrs	20–30 yrs	30–40 yrs	40–50 yrs	>50 yrs
Male	20–30	14	23	33	43	44
	>30	1	3	7	9	8
Female	25–30	12	17	21	29	34
	>30	3	5	4	9	15

BMI, Body Mass Index
Source: Anon., 1983.

Population studies that have taken this into account have shown that a part, but not all, of the differences in blood pressure between groups can be explained by differences in body mass. The effect of dietary weight reduction upon the progress of heart disease caused by **hypertension** has not been examined. A study resulting in sufficient statistical significance to demonstrate a worthwhile effect would be too costly. There have, however, been numerous studies upon the efficacy of weight loss in reducing blood pressure itself. The results have been conflicting, but the balance of evidence suggests that weight loss is accompanied by a reduction in blood pressure.

Table 6.4 — Conditions carrying increased risks associated with overweight

Gall-bladder disease
Coronary heart disease
High blood pressure (hypertension)
Increased blood lipid concentrations
Diabetes mellitus
Some cancers
Surgical operations

Obesity is closely associated with maturity onset or non-insulin-dependent diabetes mellitus (Type II diabetes – see Chapter 8). Most Type II diabetics have an upper body distribution of excess fat and enlarged fat cells. This leads to the condition of '**insulin-insensitivity**' or insulin resistance, in which the adipose tissue (and other tissues such as muscle) need more insulin to achieve a specific metabolic task (e.g. glucose transport into the cell). This, in turn, causes the pancreas to secrete more insulin, leading to high plasma concentrations of the hormone, insulin (**hyperinsulinaemia**). One effect of this is that the liver produces more very low density lipoproteins (see Chapter 7), leading to **hyperlipidaemia**. This may be one of the reasons for an observed association between upper body obesity and coronary heart disease and explains why many studies have shown no residual effect of total weight on coronary heart disease risk once age, sex, high blood pressure, increased blood cholesterol and diabetes mellitus have been taken into account.

HOW DO WE BECOME OBESE?

Our bodies need a certain amount of energy each day in order to function. Normally this would be in the range 1800–2500 kcal (7550–10 300 kJ) although different individuals require different amounts. This energy is required to sustain **resting** (or **basal**) **metabolism** which includes all the vital body chemistry, maintenance of the heart beat, respiration, maintenance of body temperature and so on (Fig. 6.2). It constitutes something like 75% of our total energy requirements. To this we must add the obligatory heat losses accompanying the breakdown of dietary proteins, carbohydrates and fats (**diet-induced thermogenesis**), any extra heat required owing to low external temperature (**cold-induced thermogenesis**) and energy required for **physical activity**.

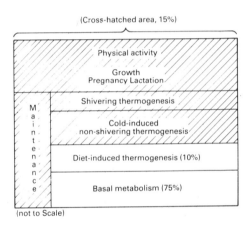

Fig. 6.2 — Human energy requirements, with percentage of total energy expenditure for a typical adult given in parenthesis.

Pregnant and lactating women have extra requirements for these energy-demanding physiological conditions and, of course, a great deal of energy is required in infancy, childhood and adolescence for growth. All this energy is normally supplied in the food we eat, but when this is not available we can use, first, the glycogen stored in the liver and, second, the fat stored in the adipose tissue. There is, therefore, a simple relationship between the food energy we eat, the energy we expend and changes in the energy stored within the body and they can be represented by a simple thermodynamic equation (see Fig. 6.3):

$$E(\text{IN}) = E(\text{OUT}) + \text{change in body energy}$$

where $E(\text{IN})$ is the energy of the food eaten, $E(\text{OUT})$ is daily heat production, and 'change in body energy' represents the change in energy value of body constituents. This is mainly the fat stores but could also be glycogen or tissue protein.

Food *energy intake* can be measured in a number of ways. Measurement of food intake is not an easy matter (see also Chapter 2). People can be asked to keep diary

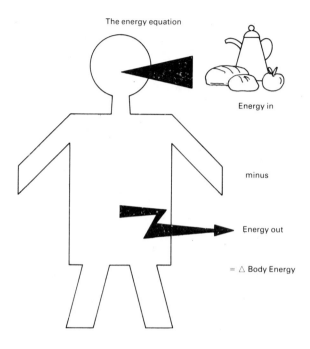

The energy equation

Energy in

minus

Energy out

$= \triangle$ Body Energy

Fig. 6.3 — The energy equation.

records of the foods they eat. This is likely to be inaccurate but is better than getting them simply to remember what they ate over a previous period of time (the Recall method), which is notoriously unreliable. More accurate is a daily **weighed intake** in which people are supplied with a balance and asked to weigh every item they consume and keep a record, usually over a seven-day period. One problem is likely to be that only the most highly motivated will keep up a reliable record, and another is that the necessity to record may itself influence food habits.

Whichever recording method is used, we will still need to translate weights of food into energy values and this is generally done using the *'McCance and Widdowson' Food Tables* (Paul and Southgate, 1978). This is now available on computer and there are programs to help convert data on weights of different foods consumed into energy intakes, with the opportunity to break down the results into values for fat, carbohydrate and protein. The most accurate system for measuring energy intake is the '**duplicate plate**' method. At every meal or snack occasion, the subject makes up a duplicate meal, exactly similar to the one eaten. The duplicate meal is then sent to the laboratory where its energy value is determined by bomb calorimetry. The proportions of the energy-yielding constituents, protein, fat and carbohydrate, can also be determined chemically. This method is infrequently used because it is time-consuming and expensive, but it is useful for occasional spot checks on the accuracy of more convenient methods.

Energy expenditure has to be measured by some form of calorimetry. There are two basic methods: **respiration (indirect) calorimetry** and **direct calorimetry**. In the first, the amounts of oxygen consumed and the amounts of carbon dioxide expired are measured, since these are related directly to heat production in the body. The measurements can be made either by using a **whole body calorimeter**, which is a special room in which the subject lives for a period of time; or more simply by the subject wearing a face mask connected to a bag, into which the expired gas is collected and from which samples can be withdrawn for analysis. In direct calorimetery, the subject stays in the whole body calorimeter, which is equipped to be able to measure directly the heat produced by the body.

We have already discussed various ways of measuring changes in the fat stores. For the purposes of fundamental research, it is possible to use animals as experimental subjects in which direct and more accurate measurements of changes in body composition can be made by carcass analysis after slaughter.

You can easily see, from the energy equation, that if the rate of consumption of food energy exceeds the rate at which the body can expend energy, the result will be an increase in body energy stores and this will almost certainly be an increase in the fat stored in adipose tissue. In the past, there have been two schools of thought concerning why people put on weight: the glutony school and the inheritance school (Table 6.5). However, it is not necessary to assume that people who become overweight have eaten more food than those who maintain ideal weight. Every person's requirements for energy are different from everyone else's. If a person has a low requirement, then he or she will need a low intake to keep the energy equation in balance.

Table 6.5 — Extremes of view on the natural history of obesity

---

The gluttony school:
Since the immediate causes of obesity are overeating and under-exercising, the remedies are available to all, but many patients require help in using them.

                                                          Davidson and Passmore (1969)

The inheritance school:
I wish to propose that obesity is an inherited disorder and due to a genetically determined defect in an enzyme; in other words, that people who are fat are born fat and nothing much can be done about it.

                                                          Astwood (1962)

While it is well known that overweight and obesity 'runs in families' it is not known whether this is due to inheritance or to a family environment in which the members are used to eating a large amount of food. We don't know much about what determines energy requirements, but there is probably a large influence of inheritance since the degree of overweight in children is much influenced by whether parents are themselves overweight, as can be seen in Table 6.6. Some strains of mice and rats have an inherited defect in their ability to 'burn off' energy that is excess to requirements, leading to a condition of gross obesity, as illustrated in Plate 6.1. Normally, animals have some ability to increase heat production in response to overfeeding. This extra heat production is thought to occur in a special type of adipose tissue called '**brown adipose tissue**' and this may be one of the ways in which the normal body maintains ideal weight in the face of overconsumption.

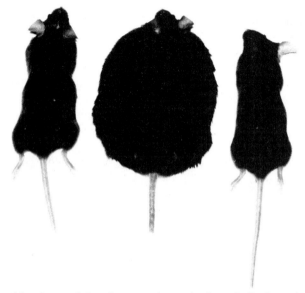

Plate 6.1 — Lean and obese litter mates in a strain of genetically obese mice.

Table 6.6 — Parental influences on the acquisition of obesity

History	Percent of obese group	Age of onsent Childhood (%)	Adult (%)
Both parents overweight	34	74	26
Mother only overweight	43	33	67
Father only overweight	3	50	50
Neither parent overweight	20	30	70

Source: Gurr *et al.*, 1982.

Human beings also have brown adipose tissue. In babies this plays an important part in temperature regulation, and Fig. 6.4 shows typical distibutions of brown adipose tissue in the bodies of newborn infants. Some people who put on weight easily may have a reduced capacity to make use of this ability of brown adipose to burn off excess calories, although this hypothesis has not been proven for human beings.

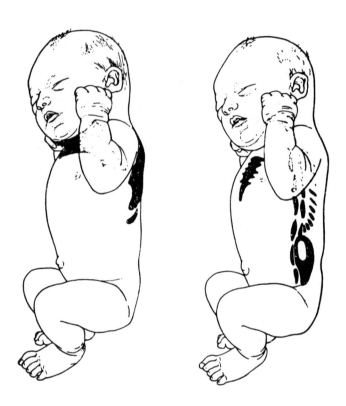

Fig. 6.4 — Typical positions of brown adipose tissue in the newborn baby. Source: Hull and Hardman, 1970.

We are equally ignorant of the factors that govern energy intake. The palatability of food is one influence. It is easier to maintain weight on a bland monotonous diet than on one which contains a variety of interesting, delicious and succulent foods all designed to tempt the appetite. This can easily be demonstrated by feeding rats with tasty human foods and comparing their growth with those fed a laboratory diet. Energy density may be another factor. If the mechanisms that control our food intake monitor bulk in some way, as seems possible, then those foods that contain more calories per unit weight will contribute to a higher energy intake. This will be particularly marked for fat-rich foods since fats contain over twice as many calories per gram as proteins or carbohydrates. In contrast, fibre-rich foods are bulky and have a low energy density, so that diets containing them are likely to contribute less to weight gain.

Food intake is also subject to control by a number of psychological factors. Thus many people tend to overeat at times of great stress or as a result of boredom. On the other hand psychological problems may cause teenage girls to reduce their energy intakes — in its severest form this can lead to a condition known as **anorexia nervosa**.

HOW DO WE LOSE WEIGHT?

Again, we need only to look at the energy equation to see that body energy stores should be reduced only when the rate of energy expenditure exceeds the rate of energy intake over a period of time.

Body energy is stored as fat, carbohydrate and protein and it should be emphasized that it is specifically the fat stored in the white adipose tissue that needs to be mobilized in a slimming regime. Adipose tissue, like all other body tissues, is composed of cells called fat cells or, more scientifically, **adipocytes**. Although these cells contain all the biochemical apparatus possessed by other cells, they are unique in being able to expand to many times their normal size to accommodate additional fat that needs to be stored. This is demonstrated in Plates 6.2 (a) and (b), which show sections through adipose tissue of a lean and an obese person, respectively.

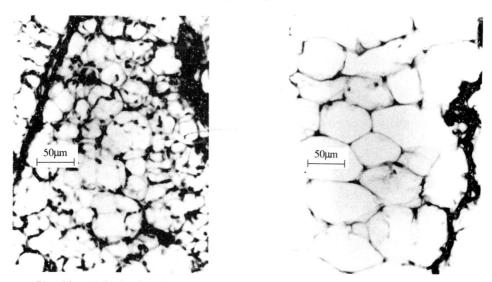

Plate 6.2 — (a) Section through adipose tissue in a lean person. (b) Section through adipose tissue in an obese person.

During slimming, fat will be lost from the fat cells and they will shrink in size. Although the main contributor to changes in the size of the fat stores is changes in the size of individual cells, a given fat store could be larger by virtue of having more cells. Fat cells begin to develop in the foetus and continue to develop in early life. During childhood, however, the maximum is reached, and further increases in the fat stores occur only by increases in the size of cells. There is some evidence in experimental animals that certain stimuli, like overfeeding or a high fat diet, can trigger off the process of cell division to create more fat cells, but there is little evidence that this generally occurs in man in normal circumstances. Indeed, the concept, once prevalent (Table 6.7), that overfeeding babies led to lifelong obesity by virtue of stimulating the production of more fat cells has now been discredited. Obese people seem to have much the same number of fat cells as normal people, no matter whether they became obese as children or as adults (Table 6.8).

Table 6.7 — The fat cell hypothesis

- Overnutrition in early life causes the production of 'excess' fat cells (hypercellularity; 'hyperplastic obesity').

- The possession of these 'excess' fat cells confers a predisposition to obesity.

Table 6.8 — Number of fat cells in adult women

	Normal	Obese	
		0–8 yrs at onset	Over 20 yrs at onset
No. of cells (x 10^9)	43.0	45.5	45.0
No. of subjects	18	24	28

Source: Gurr *et al.*, 1982.

For successful slimming, therefore, we conclude that we must either increase energy expenditure or decrease energy intake.

Energy expenditure
The most obvious way to increase energy expenditure is to increase the general level of physical activity. Some people are discouraged in their endeavours to exercise because the energy cost of various quite strenuous activities is apparently quite small. In other words, it takes a lot of activity to burn off a small amount of fat. It is much better to engage in regular moderate exercise, than in isolated and infrequent bouts of frenzied activity. Quite apart from the energy cost of the activity itself, exercise seems to stimulate diet-induced thermogenesis. There is not a lot of evidence to suggest that there are big differences in the thermic effect of different foods (i.e. the heat produced in response to the metabolism of different dietary components), but some work has indicated that obese people tend to have a poorer thermic response to overfeeding with fat than individuals who do not have weight problems.

Energy intake
Most people think of slimming in terms of reducing their food intake — generally known as dieting. We clearly need to take in less energy than we expend: how much less depends on the degree of overweight. Table 6.9 shows the average intakes of energy of

people on three dietary regimes. People who are seriously overweight are very unlikely to be able to indulge in strenuous exercise and may need a **very low calorie diet** (VLCD). Those who are slightly or moderately overweight can combine greater exercise with a correspondingly less restrictive diet.

Table 6.9 — Ranges of energy intakes appropriate to weight maintenance or loss

Diet	Energy intake	
	(kcal)	(kJ)
Normal	1800–2500	7500–10 500
For moderate weight loss	800–1500	3350–6300
Very low calorie diet (VLCD)	<600	<2500

A summary of the types of slimming diets which are available is shown in Table 6.10. These regimes will be discussed separately, since in moderate weight loss we are dealing with simple reduction in body fat and the main problem is in adhering to the diet; with VLCD we are dealing with more complex changes in metabolism and need to consider the dangers that may be associated with too rapid weight loss.

Table 6.10 — Types of slimming diet

Slimming diets involve changes in:
    the total amount of energy

and perhaps
    the composition of the diet and of foods contributing to it.

Slimming diets are categorized as:
    Low carbohydrate
    Low fat
    Calorie counting
    High fibre
    Very low calorie

Moderate weight loss
Energy expenditure, like other biological variables, is distributed about a mean so that we can expect human 'normal' expenditure to cover a broad range. This will generally be somewhere between 1800 and 2500 kcals (7550–10 500 kJ). This is the range of energy intake, therefore, which we would expect to find in people maintaining weight. Normal slimming diets would be in the range 800–1500 kcal (3350–6300 kJ) depending on energy expenditure and the weight required to be lost.

There seems to be an infinite number of ways of trying to achieve weight loss, as can be readily appreciated from the selection of books and magazines available on the subject and advertisements for new wonder slimming methods that come and go with monotonous regularity. We can conclude that none are very effective, otherwise they would presumably not be so ephemeral. Setting aside the way-out diets, such as eating nothing but pineapples or lettuce leaves, and concentrating on those with a serious scientific basis, there are two main aspects of the diets to consider:

● the total amount of energy in the diet
● the composition of the diet, and of the foods contributing to it.

One of the major benefits of dietary regimes that try to focus on eating limited amounts of a wide variety of foods, rather than prescribing specific regimes, can be that it is easier to make certain of achieving an adequate intake of all the essential nutrients. The more the intake of energy is restricted, the more likely is it that some essential nutrients will be in short supply. Since the aim of a good slimming diet is to reduce energy intake without going short on essential nutrients, we must choose foods that have a high nutrient density, that is to say they should provide large amounts of a wide variety of nutrients per unit of energy. Fig. 6.5 illustrates how different foods can differ widely in nutrient density.

One of the main reasons why attempts to lose weight and then maintain ideal weight so often fail, is the problem of motivation. Nowadays, eating is a social activity not

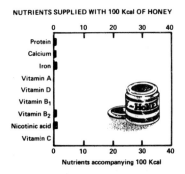

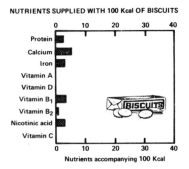

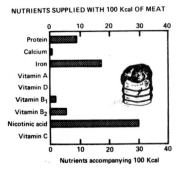

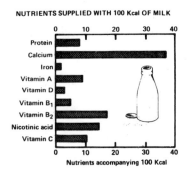

Fig. 6.5 — Nutrients supplied with 100 kcal of different foods. The figures represent the percentage of the RDA supplied with each 100 kcal of the food. From Yudkin, 1981. Reproduced with permission from Milk Industry, the International Dairy Journal.

simply a means of keeping alive. The principle behind slimming clubs is that they enable people with similar problems to learn from each other, and to be encouraged by each other and it is probably true to say that more people achieve success through slimming clubs than by tackling the task alone, or relying on advice from the family doctor. More importantly, healthy eating, whether the main motivation is for weight control or for some other health reason, is not simply a matter of following a set of dietary rules, but of changing the whole lifestyle.

A major problem in weight loss is maintaining the weight loss over a long period of time. Figs. 6.6(a) – (c) show the percentage overweight of a group of women (a) before restricted diet treatment, (b) after one year of intensive dietary treatment (when weight loss was considerable) and (c) after five years (when motivation was lost during a period without dietary supervision, and the weight increased).

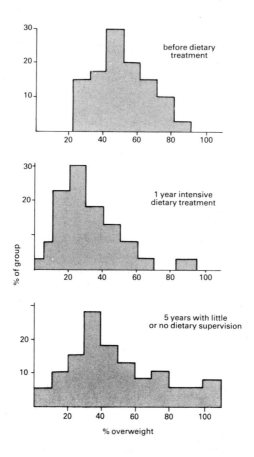

Fig. 6.6 — An illustration of the difficulty in maintaining weight loss by young obese girls without supervision. From Lloyd, 1969. Reproduced with permission from Churchill Livingstone.

Low carbohydrate diets

For a low carbohydrate diet, the slimmer is usually provided with a list of foods designated '**carbohydrate foods**' that must be avoided or severely restricted; other foods are allowed *ad libitum*. The principle behind the diet is not that carbohydrate calories are less fattening, but that people automatically reduce their intake to about 1500 kcals (6300 kJ). This type of diet was once widely advocated and part of the thinking was that if carbohydrate foods such as bread were not eaten, then this automatically restricted the energy-rich butter or jam that was associated with them. It was also claimed that fatty foods were 'self-regulating' since they induced satiety. We now know, however, that there are many people who can eat enormous quantities of fat and for whom this type of diet would not work. Furthermore, this type of diet goes against modern concepts of 'healthy' eating, which favour low fat and high carbohydrate, especially fibre, intakes (see Chapter 1).

Low carbohydrate diets can involve the elimination or reduction of 'carbohydrate' foods, as described above. Alternatively, foods are available that resemble the conventional foods except that the carbohydrate component has been reduced while retaining the same bulk of food. An example is a 'slimmer's bread' with reduced starch content, the volume being maintained by the introduction of more air into the texture of the loaf during the baking process. The idea is that the slimmer will appear to be eating the same bulk of food, but fewer calories. Other alternatives are to replace conventional carbohydrates such as starch with '**bulking agents**' or sugar with artificial sweeteners.

'Bulking agents' are usually polysaccharides, such as polydextrose, in which the sugar linkages are not hydrolysed by the digestive enzymes in the small intestine. The monosaccharides should therefore not be released and absorbed and the material should have no energy value. A problem here is that the substances pass down the gut to the large intestine, where they are degraded, at least in part, by the gut bacteria. These generate gas, causing flatulence, and volatile fatty acids, which can be absorbed and used for energy.

Recent research has shown that some of these bulking agents can have energy values as much as half that of starch. Many low calorie sweeteners rely on the fact that very small amounts with negligible energy value have much greater sweetness than the sucrose that they replace: examples are the peptide **aspartame**, the protein **thaumatin** and, of course, **saccharin**. Some sugar alcohols, such as maltitol and lactitol are sweet yet not hydrolysed by disaccharidases in the small intestine. However, the same problem exists as for bulking agents: they are degraded in the large intestine by bacteria and have a larger energy value than once supposed.

Low fat diets

For a low fat diet, the slimmer is presented with a list of high fat foods which must be avoided or severely reduced. The principle is that fat has more than twice the energy value of carbohydrate (9 kcal/g *vs* 4 kcal/g) and, therefore, represents a very dense form of energy. Low fat diets are very much in line with current dietary guidelines and are, therefore, regarded by many as beneficial in a wider sense than just weight reduction. However, diets are only successful if people are able to adhere to them for long periods, maybe a lifetime.

Fat adds palatability and enjoyment to the diet. If a diet is uninteresting and monotonous then it is very unlikely that people will be able to stick with it for very long, and this is one of the major disadvantages of such low fat regimes. The problem is being overcome by an increasing variety of low fat spreads coming on the market. These frequently have only 50% or less of the fat contained in the more traditional foods, butter and margarine. The fat content of milk can be adjusted to be nearly zero (skimmed milk) or half the fat of whole milk (semi-skimmed). Sales of reduced fat milks have risen dramatically from only 4% in 1983 to 25% in 1989. Other types of traditionally high fat foods, such as cheeses and sausages, can now be obtained in low fat varieties. There is an increasing tendency for meat animals to be reared with much reduced carcass fat compared with a few years ago.

Calorie counting diets
For a calorie counting diet, the person is allowed to eat any foods that provide a given energy intake, usually between 800 and 1500 kcals (3350–6300 kJ). This type of diet has freedom of choice, the advantage being that the slimmer can eat a varied and interesting diet, and under these conditions is likely to retain motivation for longer. There are many disadvantages. It may require weighing much of the food consumed, together with the calculation of total daily energy intake, or the purchase of foods with defined amounts of energy. These factors tend to militate against adherence to the diet. There seems to be a tendency for individuals to develop a false sense of their ability to estimate accurately the food consumed. They then stop weighing the food items and calculating their energy intake. It is a common experience for clinicians to have patients who state that they have failed to lose weight on a diet providing 1000 kcal daily (4200 kJ) but then lose weight on the same number of kcals, under strictly supervised conditions.

As in the cases of low carbohydrate and low fat diets, the slimmer on the calorie counting diet has access to a wide range of processed foods in which carbohydrate and fat components have been replaced by non-calorific components to provide the same bulk as the normal foods but with fewer calories. **Non-calorific bulking agents** are usually:

— *air*, as in calorie-reduced baked products;
— *water*, as in low calorie fat spreads, where the water is held in a water-in-oil emulsion by the use of sophisticated emulsifier technology;
— *dietary fibre*, non-starch polysaccharides etc, which provide bulk which is assumed to have negligible energy value;
— *fat analogues*, such as polyglycerol (see Fig. 6.7) or sucrose polyesters, which have fat-like texture but are not digested by lipases in the gut and therefore provide no energy.

A potential problem with these last-mentioned materials is that they may reduce the absorption of fat-soluble vitamins, and more research is needed before they are used in food manufacturing. Another type of fat that could be more extensively used is the type known as **medium chain triacylglycerols (MCT)**. Glycerides with short- and medium-chain fatty acids (less than carbon length C12) are found in milk fat and coconut oil. MCTs refined from coconut oil are used in the treatment of patients with fat malabsorption since they are not absorbed like the long-chain fatty acids which are

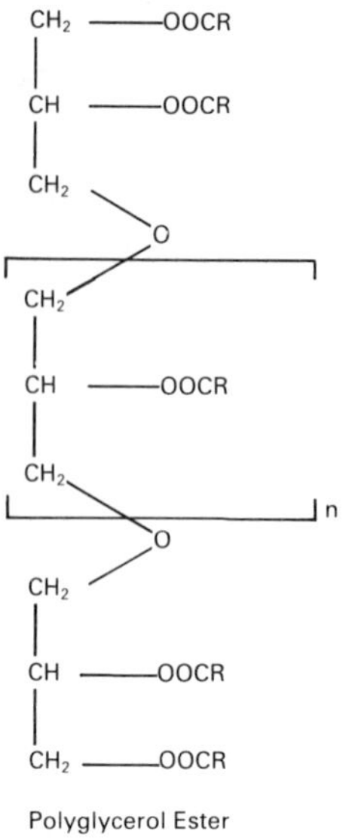

```
CH₂ ————OOCR
 |
CH  ————OOCR
 |
CH₂
       \
        O
  ┌─────/────────────────┐
  |  CH₂
  |   |
  | CH  ————OOCR
  |   |
  | CH₂
  └─────────────────────┘ n
        \
         O
  CH₂   /
   |
  CH  ————OOCR
   |
  CH₂ ————OOCR
```

Polyglycerol Ester

Fig. 6.7 — The structure of polyglycerol ester.

incorporated into the blood lipoproteins, but are absorbed as free acids into the portal bloodstream and metabolized in the liver. Long-chain fatty acids carried as lipoproteins are normally deposited in adipose tissue; short- and medium- chain acids are completely oxidized in the liver and so do not contribute to the adipose tissue mass directly. Thus, their wider use in foods could be beneficial to slimmers.

Another type of food to aid slimmers on calorie counting diets is the **complete meal** concept. These are often in the form of biscuits with a defined number of Calories (kcal) which are fortified with micronutrients and protein and are designed to cover the slimmer's complete nutritional needs. No calculations are needed, apart from reading the packet, and in theory this ought to be a reliable way of ensuring a restricted energy intake while maintaining good overall nutrition. Needless to say, the major problem is one of sheer monotony and boredom and it is very difficult for people to adhere to such a regime for long periods.

High fibre diets
High fibre dietary regimes have been brought into sharp focus by the success of Audrey Eyton's book: *The F-Plan Diet*. The philosophy is that firstly, dietary fibre has a very low intrinsic energy value compared with starch and secondly, that the bulkiness given to the diet physically limits the total amount of energy-giving foods that can be eaten. Given that many high fibre foods such as wholegrain cereals, beans, fruit and vegetables contribute useful amounts of micronutrients, such diets can be very successful and nutritious. Many, however, would find them monotonous and unpalatable and might have

great difficulty in adhering to them for very long. In addition, the efficacy of high fibre diets in reducing energy intake has not yet been satisfactorily proven.

Very low calorie diets (VLCD)

VLCDs are those that reduce daily food energy consumption to levels below 600 kcals for several consecutive days or weeks. They are recommended only for patients with severe obesity problems where less rigorous diets (800–1000 kcal) are ineffective. They should only be used under medical supervision. When energy intakes are restricted to this extent, it should be borne in mind that the body's energy expenditure adapts in two important ways. Firstly, the energy expenditure component known as **diet-induced thermogenesis** is relatively less than the 10% or so which occurs at normal energy intakes because less food is being metabolized. Secondly, basal metabolism adapts to a lower level, because at such low intakes, body energy losses occur not only from adipose tissue fat, but also from body protein. Thus, lean body mass as well as fat decreases. One of the reasons why total fasting has been virtually abandoned as therapy is because a small number of unexpected deaths occurred, attributed to losses of essential protein from certain tissues.

The development of VLCDs has sought to meet these depletion-induced changes by providing high quality protein, by formulating preparations that optimize the ratio of protein to carbohydrate and by including the complete range of minerals and vitamins. Protein is required to minimize the losses in tissue nitrogen that occur at low energy intakes; carbohydrate is necessary to maintain insulin secretion and it also seems to assist in the conservation of proteins and minerals. Some fat is needed to maintain intake of essential fatty acids, linoleic and linolenic acids.

CONCLUSION

Obesity is the storage of excess dietary energy as fat in adipose cells found in many parts of the body. Life assurance company data are used by nutritionists to construct graphs relating weight, height and life expectancy, so that an ideal range of weight-for-height can be determined. Many people in the UK are overweight according to these and other criteria, and statistics show a large proportion of the population is overweight. Excessive overweight or obesity is related to increased risk of a number of diseases of affluence, such as coronary heart disease and diabetes.

The interest in reducing weight is evident from the large number of books and magazines sold on slimming. Indeed, a very high proportion of the community is said to be on a reducing diet at any time. Much advice abounds, and most of it misinforms the public. There is no easy way to lose weight, as, for a loss in weight, energy intake must be cut down to below energy expenditure, so that body fat can be used as an energy source and its quantity reduced. There is no alternative to this and, therefore, voluntary weight reduction always requires application of will power. None of the faddist diets recommended are effective in the long term: it is better to reduce overall intake to about half the energy value of the habitual diet, ensuring that a variety of foods is consumed. Motivation can be maintained by self-help groups like slimming clubs. Very low calorie diets are recommended only when a person has a severe obesity problem and other less rigorous diets are ineffective. They should only be given under strict medical supervision.

REFERENCES

Anon. (1983) Obesity: A Report of the Royal College of Physicians. *Journal of the Royal College of Physicians of London*, **17** (1).

Anon. (1986) *Diet, nutrition and health*. British Medical Association, London.

Davidon, S. and Passmore, R. (1969) *Human nutrition and dietetics*. 4th ed. Churchill Livingstone, Edinburgh.

DHSS (1987) *The use of Very Low Calorie Diets in obesity*. Report on Health and Social Subjects No. 31. HMSO, London.

Eyton, A. (1982) *The F-plan diet*. Penguin Books Ltd, Harmondsworth, Middlesex, UK.

Festing, M. F. W. (ed.) (1979) *Animal models of obesity*. Macmillan Publishing Co, New York.

Garrow, J. S. (1978) *Energy balance and obesity in man*, 2nd ed. Elsevier-North Holland, London.

Gurr, M.I., Jung, R.T., Robinson, M.P. and James, W.P.T. (1982) Adipose tissue cellularity in man: the relationship between fat cell size and number, the mass and distribution of body fat and the history of weight gain or loss. *International Journal of Obesity*, **6**, 419–436.

Hull, D. and Hardman, M.J. (1970) Brown adipose tissue in newborn mammals. In: Lindberg, O. (ed.) *Brown adipose tissue*. American Elsevier, New York.

Lloyd, J. (1969) In: McLean, B. I. and Howard, A. N. (eds) *Obesity: medical and scientific aspects*. E & S Livingstone, Edinburgh.

Paul, A. A. and Southgate, D. A. T. (1978) *McCance and Widdowson's The composition of foods*. 4th ed. MRC Special Report Series No. 297. HMSO, London.

Rothwell, N. J. and Stock, M. J. (1979) A role for brown adipose tissue in diet induced thermogenesis. *Nature* **281**, 31–35.

Stern, M. P. and Haffner S. M. (1986) Body fat distribution and hyperinsulinaemia as risk factors for diabetes and cardiovascular disease. *Arteriosclerosis*, **6**, 123–130.

Yudkin, J. (1981) Milk – the uniquely nutritious food, Milk Industry, **Nov.**, 18–23

7

Diet and coronary heart disease
Ann Walker

Introduction

Coronary heart disease (CHD) and hypertension (high blood pressure) are the two most common disorders of the cardiovascular system in Britain and many industrialized countries today. They are much less common in rural communities in the Third World, although increasing in incidence among the wealthy of these countries. The role of dietary factors in the development (aetiology) and treatment of CHD has been the subject of much study and still remains contentious, despite the fact that one of the principal methods of treatment of the disease is by dietary restriction or modification.

DESCRIPTION OF CORONARY HEART DISEASE

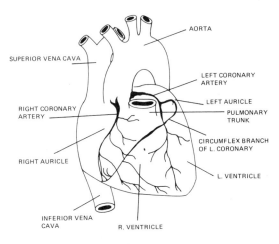

ANTERIOR SURFACE OF THE HEART

Fig. 7.1 — Interior surface of the heart.

Fig. 7.1 shows a diagram of the heart and its blood supply. Although the heart pumps blood around the body, the muscle tissue does not have access to this blood. The heart is supplied with its own arteries, the coronary arteries, which arise from the aorta. As can be seen in the diagram, there is a left and a right coronary artery and to some extend their functions overlap, in that some tissue is serviced by both arteries. This can be an important feature of recovery from heart attacks, depending on exactly where in the heart tissue damage occurs.

Coronary heart disease or CHD is also called **ischaemic heart disease**. The disease is a group of syndromes arising from the failure of the coronary arteries to supply sufficient blood to the myocardium or heart tissue. In most cases the disease is associated with **atherosclerosis** (furring up) of the coronary arteries. Apart from sudden death, **myocardial infarction** or **angina pectoris** can result.

Myocardial infarction: **necrosis** (death of tissue) of part of the heart muscle due to failure of the blood supply (ischaemia). This can cause sudden death; or damaged tissue may heal, leaving a scar. Recovery depends on the severity of the damage (lesion). Infarction is usually initiated by a **thrombus** (blood clot) forming in an atherosclerotic coronary artery. This may dislodge and pass down the artery until it finds the lumen (space in centre of artery) too small to pass and then it gets stuck. The artery, which may already be partly blocked (occluded) with atheroslerosis, then becomes completely blocked and blood ceases to flow along it, depriving heart muscle tissue of oxygen and nutrients.

Angina pectoris: pain in the chest (or sometimes so-called referred pain in the left arm) brought on by exercise. People with this have reduced blood flow to the heart owing to atherosclerosis and must avoid sudden exercise. People with angina are at greater risk of a heart attack.

It is important to remember that CHD has two distinct stages: atherosclerosis and thrombosis. The former is slow in development, while the latter can be sudden and precipitate a 'heart attack'. The development of each stage is influenced differently by diet, as indicated later in this chapter.

RISK FACTORS IN CHD IDENTIFIED FROM EPIDEMIOLOGY

The role of epidemiology in the study of human nutrition has already been described in Chapters 1 and 5, but will be discussed again here because of the particularly important role it has to play in the study of CHD. In using this technique, populations suffering from high rates of CHD can be compared with those that have very little. These data can then be correlated with various lifestyle factors, including diet.

In **retrospective** epidemiological studies, dietary information is collected from people who have already had CHD. The method is not satisfactory as the patients available for questioning are only those who survive CHD and, in addition, are those who come into hospital. There is also difficulty in matching with controls in the community retrospectively. The best way to conduct epidemiological studies is to use **prospective** studies. In these studies, people are recruited into the study as healthy individuals, and then their lifestyle, diet and disease patterns are monitored over time. Some will and some will not go on to develop CHD. Those that do not, act as the control population.

Some fifty years ago CHD was a disease of older men of the well-to-do classes. However, between 1950 and 1965 there was a huge increase in CHD in Britain and other countries, with other social classes affected. It was particularly striking that cases were occurring more and more among the age group 35–44 years, in addition to the older age groups. From 1966 to 1975 figures for mortality from CHD remained high with only slight changes, including a small rise in women, who overall have a much lower incidence than men. By the time the COMA (1984) Report on *Diet and Cardiovascular Disease* was published, the levels had reached a maximum and there was little evidence that the rate was falling. Some people have called CHD a 'modern epidemic'. The percentage contribution of CHD to overall figures for death among men and women in the UK can be seen in Fig. 7.2.

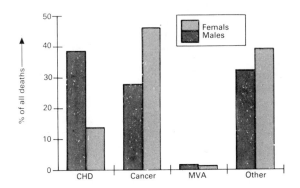

Fig 7.2 — Contribution of CHD to overall death rate for men and women aged 40–59 years in the UK. (MVA, Motor vehicle accidents.) (Data from COMA, 1984.)

Fig. 7.3 shows the CHD mortality rate per 100 000 of the population in the 1980s in various countries. More recently, the rate of CHD in some western countries such as Finland and USA has declined markedly, while the rate in Britain continues to be high. There is as yet only a very slight indication that the rate is coming down in Britain and that is among men of the professional classes. The inertia in public health education and lack of a clear policy has cost the UK dear. However, it is by no means obvious why previous world leader countries mentioned above, have achieved such a rapid decline in rate. Greater awareness of a whole range of dietary and lifestyle risk factors (discussed below) may well contribute, but it is unlikely that any single factor is responsible.

Within the UK there are geographic distributions of risk, with Scotland and Northern Ireland very high risk areas. Despite differences in the incidence of CHD in different countries, there is no evidence of racial immunity to the disease. This is exemplified by

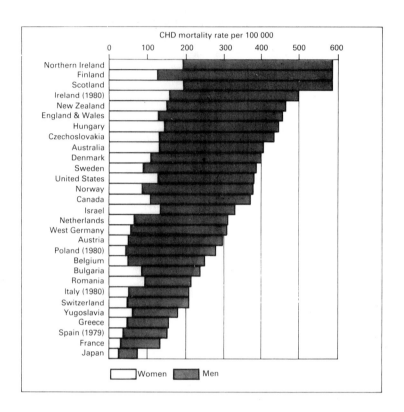

Fig. 7.3 — Coronary heart disease mortality rates for men and women aged 40 - 69. Age
standardized rates per 100000 for 1987 unless otherwise stated. Copyright 1990 OVEU Dundee
University. (Kindly supplied by Professor H. Tunstall-Pedoe.)

the incidence of CHD among the Japanese. While the levels in Japan are low, those
Japanese living in California show a rate 10 times higher.

The whole gamut of risk factors which have been implicated in the aetiology of CHD
have already been discussed in Chapter 1, but Table 7.1 lists those most often cited.

The most famous prospective epidemiological study in CHD is that of Framingham,
Ma., USA which is also the longest on-going programme. (In 1949, 5000 healthy men
and women over 30 years old were taken into the study. Records were made of their way
of life, illnesses etc., and they were medically examined every two years.) Now there are
some 20 other prospective studies in progress throughout the world. In all the studies
which have so far reported, it has been shown that the three principle risk factors for
CHD are a high plasma (or serum) total cholesterol (hypercholesterolaemia), high
arterial blood pressure (hypertension) and cigarette smoking. Table 7.2 shows
the increased risk identified for these factors in two of the major prospective
epidemiological studies.

Table 7.1 — Some risk factors in coronary heart disease

General
● Maleness
● Increasing age
● A family history of CHD
Body Status
● <u>Hypercholesterolaemia</u>
● <u>Hypertension</u>
● Diabetes
● Obesity
Cultural/Environmental
● Diet
● <u>Cigarette Smoking</u>
● Lack of exercise
Less well demonstrated
● Stress
● Large coffee intake
● Soft drinking water

Primary risk factors are underlined in the table.

Table 7.2 — Increased risk of a heart attack in 'high risk' men in two prospective epidemiological studies

	Relative Risk	
Risk factor	Framingham (1976)	Pooling (1978)
Serum cholesterol	x 1.75 (*> 7.9 mmol/l*)	x 2.4 (*> 7.1 mmol/l*)
Blood pressure (diastolic)	x 2.2 (*> 105 mm Hg*)	x 2.2 (*>94 mm Hg*)
Smoking (cigarettes)	x 1.9 (*20/day*)	x 3.2 (*≥ 20/day*)
Aggregate risk	x 8.5	x 8.7

Another famous epidemiological study is the Seven Countries Study set up by Professor Ancel Keys (Shaper, 1988). This was based on prospective studies of men aged 40–59 years in Finland, Greece, Italy, Japan, the Netherlands, the USA and Yugoslavia. The study has shown that mean serum cholesterol level is a key factor in determining risk from CHD (Fig. 7.4).

One of the problems with blood cholesterol level is that it is, perhaps, the most

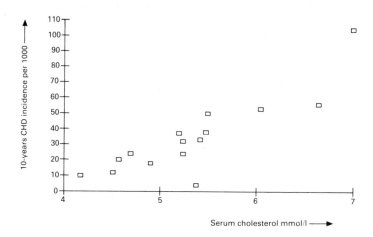

Fig. 7.4 — Relationship between serum cholesterol level and CHD from the Seven Countries Study. (Modified from Shaper, 1988.)

variable parameter which can be measured in the human body, with values for one individual varying very widely from that of the next. Such large variations are not normally seen for other biochemical measurements on blood, as limits for most parameters are narrow owing to the existence of homeostatic mechanisms. Fig. 7.5 shows the variation of serum cholesterol level of healthy male medical students in the USA. Various authorities give different levels above which there is increased risk of coronary heart disease; these range from about 4.7 to 5.3 mmol/l.

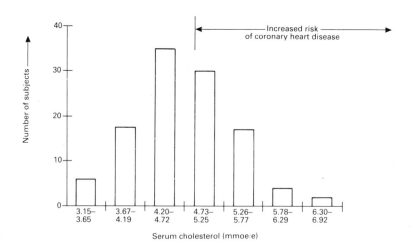

Fig. 7.5 — The variation of serum cholesterol in male medical students in the USA. (Modified from Connor and Connor, 1972.)

When populations around the world are compared, the mean plasma cholesterol levels range from about 110–280 mg/dl (2.9–7.4 mmol/l) in healthy people. Mean values in industrialized countries are much higher than those in Third World countries such as India, and the incidence of CHD is, of course, very much higher in the industrialized western world. However, the mere finding of a such a relationship between high plasma cholesterol levels and increased incidence of CHD does not mean that high cholesterol levels are causative (see Chapter 1) as epidemiological evidence can never be used as proof of cause, as so many factors vary between communities. Other evidence would therefore be sought in the quest for the cause of CHD in the form of data from animal experiments and clinical trials (see below).

Another piece of evidence to link high cholesterol levels with the incidence of coronary heart disease is that patients who have familial (inherited) hypercholesterolaemia are much more at risk of CHD. Indeed the risk of CHD caused by atherosclerosis is much reduced when plasma cholesterol remains below 4.7 mmol/l over the lifetime of an individual.

PATHOLOGY OF CORONARY HEART DISEASE: ATHEROSCLEROSIS

The pathological basis of CHD is atherosclerosis in one or both coronary arteries. It is usually associated with atherosclerosis of the aorta and other major arteries. Atherosclerosis is the formation of plaque on the inside of the major arteries, and particularly at points where they bend or branch. There are three particular sites in the body which are prone to the development of atherosclerosis. These are in the coronary arteries, the cerebral arteries (can lead to stroke) and the femoral artery (can reduce blood flow to the leg muscles and feet, causing cramp on walking).

It is customary to separate the lesions of atherosclerosis into fatty streaks, plaques and complicated lesions. Human beings are particularly prone to atherosclerosis — more so than most species, although they share this characteristic with other primates and elephants! Fig. 7.6 shows the stages in the development of atherosclerosis, and no human escapes all these stages. At around the age of 11 most people have fatty streaks, and by the age of 20 most in an affluent society have Stage 2. It is a sobering thought that a very high proportion of the young Americans in their early 20s killed in the Vietnam war showed substantial (up to 60%) occlusion (blockage) of their arteries owing to atherosclerosis.

Atherosclerosis may not necessarily be progressive, however, and unless the condition progresses to Stages 3 and 4 it will remain asymptomless. Streaks may be reversible or may proceed to plaques. Plaques are raised, soft or fibrous, established lesions of atherosclerosis, up to 1 cm in diameter. They may progress to complicated lesions due to the loss of the endothelium with surface ulceration. Fibrin is attracted to such surfaces as well as platelets and thrombosis may result.

HYPERLIPIDAEMIAS AND CHD

The relationship between plasma cholesterol and CHD has been shown in all prospective studies. It is one of the best established relationships in the epidemiology of CHD. However, association does not prove cause and effect.

Elevated levels of cholesterol and triacylglycerols (triglycerides) in the blood give rise

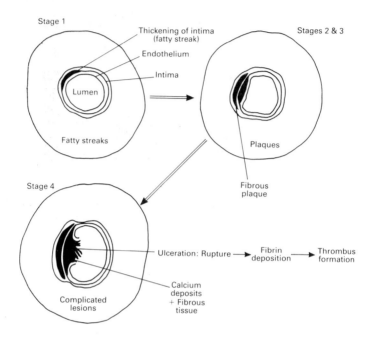

Fig. 7.6 — Stages in arterial atherosclerosis.

to a condition known as hyperlipidaemia or hyperlipoproteinaemia. Hypertriglyceridaemia, in the absence of an elevation of serum cholesterol level has not been shown to be pathogenic for atherosclerosis. However, both cholesterol and triacylglycerols are transported together in the blood in **lipoprotein** form, and frequently hypertriglyceridaemia is accompanied by hypercholesterolaemia. From a practical point of view in treatment and also because of the lack of evidence about the role of raised levels of triglycerides, serum cholesterol is used to assess risk and the efficacy of management of those at risk.

The composition of the various lipoproteins of blood plasma is shown in Fig. 7.7. The formation of these lipoproteins enables the transportation of polar lipids in the non-polar, water-based, medium of the blood. This is facilitated by coating the lipid molecule clusters with special proteins called **apoproteins** with detergent-like activity (possessing both polar and non-polar characteristics), which present a polar 'face' to the blood plasma. Each lipoprotein class has different types and/or proportions of the various apoproteins.

An overview of cholesterol metabolism and the role of the various lipoproteins in transporting cholesterol are shown in Fig. 7.8. Fig. 7.8 also shows an overview of the body's own synthesis of cholesterol in the liver. The step from acetyl coenzyme A is rate'limiting in the pathway and the action of the enzyme seems to be suceptible to inhibition or promotion by dietary means. Large amounts of saturated fatty acid in the diet promote the body to make more cholesterol.

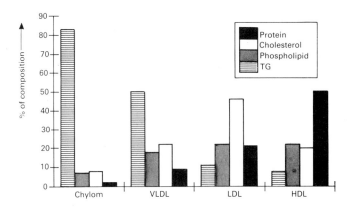

Fig. 7.7 — Composition of human serum lipoprotein classes. (Chylom, chylomicron; HDL, high density lipoprotein; LDL, low density lipoprotein; TG, triacylglycerol; VLDL, very low density lipoprotein.

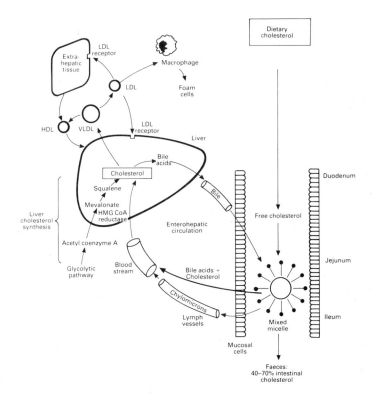

Fig. 7.8 — Cholesterol metabolism and transport by plasma lipoproteins. (Abbreviations as Fig. 7.7.)
Figure prepared by Neuza Brunoro-Costa.

The chylomicrons transport fat from the intestine to the rest of the body and finally to the liver. In fact, fat absorption occurs in two ways: some is absorbed into the blood vessels in the small intestine and then goes via the hepatic portal vein direct to the liver, and some is absorbed into the lymph system. Transport via the hepatic portal vein only occurs for some medium-chain (10 − 12 carbons or less) free fatty acids and monoacylglycerols.

Other fatty acids and diacylglycerols are taken up by the mucosal cells and resynthesized to form triacylglycerols. These are formed into spherical **chylomicrons** by the addition of phospholipids, cholesterol, cholesterol esters and a specific protein, **apoprotein B**. Thus, lipids which have been hydrolysed, resynthesized and protein-coated enter the circulation via the lymph system as chylomicrons. The lymph system delivers the chylomicrons to the blood plasma in the thoracic duct. A few hours after a large, fatty meal the chylomicrons are particularly high and can cause the plasma to take on a cloudy, rather than the normal clear appearance. The levels of chylomicrons in the blood are therefore related to the intake of fat in the diet of the immediate past, and will vary enormously from one time to another in any individual.

The function of the other plasma lipoproteins is to transport lipid material within the body. Most triacylglycerol is carried in the **very low density lipoprotein** fraction (VLDL). The **low density lipoproteins** (LDL) carry most of the cholesterol (usually 2/3 to 3/4 of the total) and the level of LDL cholesterol correlates well with total plasma cholesterol. Thus LDL cholesterol is positively related to CHD in epidemiological studies. On the other hand, despite the fact that **high density lipoproteins** (HDL) carry cholesterol, their level is negatively correlated to CHD. It is thought that HDL probably helps to mobilize cholesterol deposits from the tissues and transport them to the liver and for this reason its HDL function is sometime called 'reverse cholesterol transport'. The relative immunity of women to CHD may be due to the elevating effect of oestrogens on HDL.

The lipoproteins in a person's blood can be separated by applying a sample of the plasma to paper or gel electrophoresis. Fig. 7.9 includes the electrophoretic pattern of people with 'normal' and abnormal blood pictures.

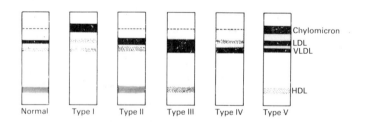

Figure 7.9 — Electrophoresis patterns of plasma from normal and hyperlipoproteinaemic patients.

The classes of hyperlipidaemia which are associated with diet are Types II and IV (Fig. 7.9). These account for the majority of cases of raised lipid blood levels. Some of

It is estimated that only a small minority (5%) of people have severe hyperlipidaemia which is primarily based upon genetic and not upon environmental factors. However, while their condition is not primarily caused by diet, their treatment always involves dietary therapy as a first approach. The type of hyperlipidaemia primarily produced by diet is referred to as exogenous or environmental, because the serum cholesterol can be reduced to 5.8 mmol/l or below by the use of diet alone and because the diet appears to be the predominant factor in the development of the condition. In all these descriptions of hyperlipidaemia (exogenous or genetic) there are obviously gradations and therefore there may not be rigid demarcations.

THE EXPERIMENTAL APPROACH IN CHD RESEARCH

The experimental approach to CHD is basically the same as that for all other branches of nutrition (see Chapter 3), and makes use of:

- Epidemiological studies
- *In vitro* studies
- Animal studies
- Clinical studies/Human trials

In trying to understand the vast literature on the subject of diet and CHD, with its claims and counterclaims, it is important always to bear in mind the type of evidence which is being examined. In the study of nutrition and its affects on health, epidemiology has an important role to play in pinpointing possible relationships which should then require further testing. Further testing can be done for some nutritional studies *in vitro*, but these studies are limited and the data are subject to variable interpretation. The next level of approach would be to find an animal model, which closely resembles man — at least for the physiological system under study. The best evidence of all (and, therefore, this carries more weight) is to undertake a controlled experiment in man. These are often called human or clinical trials.

While epidemiology gives relatively weak evidence for a causal link, say between the state of nutrition and the presence of disease, it is also powerful in the following sense. If there is no epidemiological evidence for a relationship suggested, then it is hard, even with the most refined hypothesis, backed by biochemical evidence from animal experiments and perhaps even controlled human trials, to establish such a relationship. A good example of that is that in some studies (animal and human) high levels of sucrose in the diet have been shown to raise plasma triacylglycerol levels. Suggestions have therefore been made that high levels of sucrose in the diet may predispose to CHD. But there is no epidemiological evidence for this.

Much has been made in recent years of the causal relationship between saturated fat in the diet and CHD, but the issue still remains a contentious one. The main reason for this is that there has been no controlled clinical trial of the effect of decreasing dietary intake of saturated fatty acids on the incidence of CHD. The reason is that such a trial would mean controlling people's intake, perhaps over decades. Apart from the expense of such a trial, the restriction imposed on individual freedom for many people would be unethical. However, it is the lack of such data which has caused doubts to be raised concerning the central or even unique place of saturated fat in the diet in causing CHD.

Apart from the fact that CHD, like some other diseases of affluence, is multifactorial in origin, another major problem in the study of the links between diet and CHD is the wide range of individual responses which humans show. Thus on a high saturated fat diet some individuals will and some will not develop CHD. There will be in any population those who are high responders with high cholesterol levels who are prone to CHD and those that are low responders. This is not unique to humans, however, as animals models also show this wide range of variation in blood cholesterol level in response to diets high in saturated fat. As far as animal studies are concerned, there is no ideal animal model available for the study of CHD. Most animals do not develop atherosclerosis as readily as man. Primates would be the animal of choice, but are not usually used for reasons of expense and difficulties in handling. Perhaps the pig provides the best compromise model. However, pigs are expensive to use in experiments, so the data using them are limited. The favoured animal model is still the rat, although direct comparisons with the human condition are tenuous.

THE IMPORTANCE OF HIGH BLOOD CHOLESTEROL LEVEL AS A RISK FACTOR IN CHD

Despite continuing controversy regarding the interpretation of data from epidemiological and animal studies, an important point emerges: a raised serum cholesterol concentration is essential to the development of atherosclerosis. Studies of the Japanese and other human populations show that symptomatic atherosclerosis does not frequently develop unless the mean plasma cholesterol level of the population is greater than about 4.1 mmol/l, despite the existence of hypertension. However, with even slightly raised cholesterol levels, the effect of high blood pressure is potent in increasing the risk of CHD, and this risk increases considerably if both plasma cholesterol levels and blood pressure are high (see Fig. 7.10). It is hypothesized that high blood pressure encourages blood cholesterol to be deposited in the arteries, causing atherosclerosis.

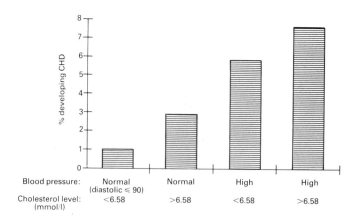

Fig. 7.10 — Interrelationships between raised serum cholesterol levels and hypertension as risk factors in the development of coronary heart disease (CHD).

pressure are high (see Fig. 7.10). It is hypothesized that high blood pressure encourages blood cholesterol to be deposited in the arteries, causing atherosclerosis.

An alternative hypothesis for the development of atherosclerosis is that the lining of the arteries becomes damaged as a result of abrasive flow of blood and (possibly) the presence of toxic oxidants in the blood (see antioxidant hypothesis below). However, in animals, even if the lining of an artery is damaged, it will not become atherosclerotic unless the animal is hypercholesterolaemic.

Clinial studies in subjects with hyperlipoproteinaemias provide some of the most direct and convincing evidence for the role of cholesterol in the aetiology of CHD. Homozygotes for familial hypercholesterolaemia carry a nearly universal risk of death from premature atherosclerosis, many dying within the first or second decade of life. In contrast, individuals having genetically determined low LDL or high HDL concentrations have been shown to have increased longevity. Clearly there is much evidence to suggest a major role for hypercholesterolaemia in the determination of CHD risk, but it is still not possible to evaluate the magnitude of this risk independently of that from other risk factors.

If raised cholesterol levels are associated with increased risk of CHD, then the question which then arises is, 'Does a reduction in cholesterol level lower the risks of CHD?' The most definitive work to date has been that of the Lipid Research Clinics Trial in the USA, early in the 1980s, in which a group of middle-aged men with high cholesterol levels took the cholesterol-lowering drug cholestyramine, which reduced their total serum cholesterol by an average of 8.5%. The implications of this study for the management of people with hypercholesterolaemia were summarized in an editorial in the *Lancet* (1984) 'These new results strongly suggest than energetic cholesterol reduction can reduce the risk of CHD perhaps by up to a half.'

The weight of evidence, some of which is summarized above, leads the majority of nutritionists (consensus view) to regard high cholesterol levels as germane to the development of CHD. Therefore, dietary modification is, in general, aimed at reducing blood cholesterol level, with a view to reducing risk of CHD.

Effects of diet, particularly on plasma cholesterol level

Table 7.3 — Some correlations between mortality rates from CHD in men (55–59 years) and the intake of certain dietary components

Positive:	Animal protein	0.78
	Cholesterol	0.76
	Meat	0.70
	Total fat	0.68
	Eggs	0.67
	Total calories	0.63
	Animal fat	0.63
None:	Fish	0.01
	Vegetable fat	0.01
	Vegetables	0.01
Negative:	Starch	-0.46
	Vegetable protein	-0.40

Source: Conner & Conner, 1972.

Overall indications of the effects of diet on mortality from CHD, taken from epidemiological data, can be seen in Table 7.3.

Although universal acceptance of the role of diet in the aetiology of CHD is still lacking, we are on much firmer ground when discussing the effects of dietary components on blood cholesterol levels. Here the data are taken from clinical trials and provide scientific fact. Dietary components that chiefly lower cholesterol do so by lowering LDL cholesterol level. Dietary fat, for example has very little effect on HDL, which contributes some 1.0–1.3 mmol/l to plasma cholesterol. There is much less cholesterol in VLDL and chylomicrons, so these lipoproteins are not of any particular note with respect to cholesterol level.

As well as, or rather than, lowering blood cholesterol levels, some foods may have beneficial effects in reducing risk of coronary heart disease for other reasons. These effects are primarily to lower blood pressure and/or to reduce the risk of thrombosis. Although the effects of foods on plasma cholesterol level is mainly discussed below, where there is evidence of CHD risk reduction due to reduction in these other factors this is mentioned.

Dietary cholesterol and plant sterols
Epidemiological evidence taken from different countries suggests that dietary intake of cholesterol is related to death rate from CHD (Fig. 7.11).

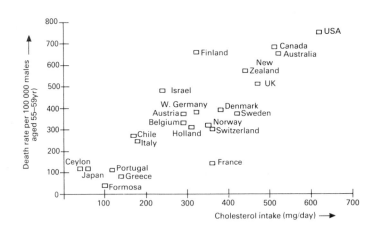

Figure 7.11 — Death rate from CHD and mean daily intake of cholesterol in diet, according to country. (Modified from Connor and Connor, 1989.)

However, although this relationship can be shown between countries, it cannot be shown within countries. Thus the Framingham study indicated that for Americans there was no correlation between the intake of dietary cholesterol and the development of CHD. However, the intakes of all the people in that study were very high. 93% of the

men consumed more than 400 mg/day of cholesterol and worldwide comparisons of
dietary cholesterol intakes indicate that this level would be associated with considerable
atherosclerotic disease. It appears from data such as those presented in Fig. 7.12 that at
higher levels of cholesterol intake, the responsiveness of serum cholesterol to a given
increase in dietary cholesterol is less pronounced than at lower intakes. However, there
is no plateau at which dietary cholesterol no longer influences serum cholesterol, as is
often supposed.

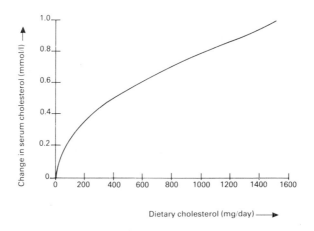

Fig. 7.12 — Predicted change in serum cholesterol in relation to dietary cholesterol. (Modified
from Vergroesen and Crawford, 1989.)

It has been suggested that because of the lack of direct relationship between
cholesterol intake and increase in serum cholesterol (Fig. 7.12) that the strong correlation
between dietary cholesterol and CHD (Fig. 7.11) may be due to dietary cholesterol acting
as an indicator of a rich diet (i.e. one high in saturated fat) rather than being causative of
the high incidence of CHD itself. If this is the case then it is, perhaps, not surprising to
find that similar patterns between dietary cholesterol intake and CHD incidence and
saturated fat intake and CHD incidence prevail between and within countries (see
below).

That the significance of high levels of dietary cholesterol in raising blood cholesterol
is regarded differently by various experts is well illustrated by the dietary guidelines in
various countries. In the USA there is strong advice to reduce dietary cholesterol, while
in the UK it tends to be played down and saturated fat given a much more prominant
role. Indeed, in the UK (COMA, 1984), dietary cholesterol has been ascribed a much
less prominent role than saturated fat. However, dietary cholesterol does have some
plasma cholesterol elevating effect and people with raised cholesterol levels would be
advised to avoid too many eggs, liver and kidneys, which are exceptionally rich sources
(see Table 7.4).

Table 7.4 — Cholesterol content of average servings of selected common foods

Food	Quantity	Cholesterol (mg)
Milk, skimmed (ml)	250	4
Cheese, cheddar (g)	30	32
Milk, whole (ml)	250	34
Tuna fish (g)	100	65
Chicken breast (g)	100	69
Beef (g)	100	88
Shrimp (g)	100	153
Egg	1 yolk	274
Liver (g)	100	435
Kidney (g)	100	800
Brains (g)	100	2000

Cholesterol is only present in animal products. Plant foods contain plant sterols, of which β-sitosterol is the best known and this, taken in large pharmaceutical doses (3 x 3–6 g per day), lowers plasma cholesterol level in man. It probably acts by competitive inhibition of cholesterol absorption or reabsorption. As the content in most foods is much below the pharmaceutical dose, it is unlikely that dietary plant sterols would exert much effect on blood cholesterol levels.

Total dietary fat
Although one of the main recommendations in the dietary guidelines is to reduce the fat content of the diet, some experts have argued that this is not justified by the experimental data. Indeed, in Chapter 5 it was pointed out by Dr Hugh Sinclair that the traditional diet of Eskimos contains the highest levels of fat intake in the world, and yet they have relatively little heart disease or other degenerative disease. He pointed out that despite the high intake of fat, the proportion of PUFA (polyunsaturated) fat was high.

Other human groups which are often quoted are the Greeks and the Japanese. In 1978, the life expectancies of both of these populations were among the highest in the world, and yet their fat intakes were very different. Greeks eat 30–40 % of their energy as fat (about the same as the British), while the Japanese only 10%. However, both have a P/S ratio (polyunsaturates:saturates) of about 1.0, compared with 0.2–0.3 for the British.

Worries about possible carcinogenic effects of PUFA have inhibited the various committees who have drawn up dietary guidelines from making more positive recommendations to increase PUFA in the diet. This and other points are discussed in the following two sections.

Saturated fats
Comparisons of epidemiological data between countries show a direct relationship between saturated fatty acid intake and mortality from CHD, as illustrated by Fig. 7.13, taken from the Seven Countries Study. However, rather like the intake of dietary

cholesterol (see above) no relationship can be shown within countries. Not surprisingly, the relationship between dietary saturated fat and the level of serum cholesterol was also shown in the Seven Countries Study. Beyond epidemiological studies, factual evidence to link saturated fat and coronary heart disease comes from animal and clinical studies. Studies in primates show that diets high in saturated fats can lead to cholesterol-rich atherosclerotic lesions of the coronary arteries. Also in animals, thrombosis may be increased by saturated fat in the diet, while PUFAs tend to decrease it. Clinical studies show that saturated fat in the diet increases blood cholesterol levels, whereas PUFAs reduce it (Table 7.5).

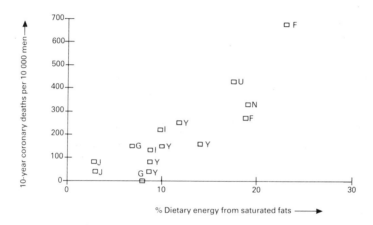

Figure 7.13 — 10-year coronary death rate of men in the Seven Countries Study in relation to percentage dietary energy from saturated fat. (F, Finland; G, Greece; I, Italy; J, Japan; N, Netherlands; U, USA; Y, Yugoslavia. (Modified from Shaper, 1988.)

Table 7.5 — Effects of dietary fatty acids on plasma cholesterol and triacylglycerols in clinical trials

Fatty acid		Cholesterol	Triacylglycerols
Medium-chain	$C_{8:0}$-$C_{10:0}$	0	↑
Lauric	$C_{12:0}$	↑	0
Myristic	$C_{14:0}$	↑↑	0
Palmitic	$C_{16:0}$	↑↑	0
Stearic	$C_{18:0}$	?↑	↑
Oleic	$C_{18:1}$	?0	0
Linoleic	$C_{18:2}$	↓	↓
Other polyunsaturated		↓	?

Polyunsaturated fats and the P/S ratio

The effect of PUFAs in reducing thrombosis was dealt with in Chapter 5, and their effect in lowering blood cholesterol has already been mentioned (Table 7.5). Epidemiological evidence shows that there is an inverse relationship between blood or fat cell content of linoleic acid and coronary heart disease, both within and between countries (Chapter 5). Linoleic acid is the most common PUFA in our diets, being high in oilseeds and in edible oils extracted from them, and is the PUFA which is most likely to increase if dietary advice to replace fats high in saturated fats with those high in PUFA is followed.

A suggestion that PUFAs increase the incidence of cancer of the bowel (colo-rectal cancer) in animal experiments led to caution being exercised in promoting the use of excess oils and fats containing PUFA and the cautious statement in the COMA Report (1984):

> There are no specific recommendations for change in the consumption of polyunsaturated and monounsaturated fatty acids, but to facilitate the recommendation for saturated fatty acids we recommend that the ratio of polyunsaturated fatty acids to saturated fatty acids (the P/S ratio) may be increased to approximately 0.45.

In fact, the animal experiments concerned have been criticized as being poorly designed (Vegroesen and Crawford, 1989), with the control group (against which the test group is compared) being deficient in essential nutrients (vitamins, essential fatty acids etc.), leading not only to inhibition of growth, but to inhibition of tumour growth (it is well known that undernutrition retards tumour growth).

In one of these experiments, a chemical carcinogen was fed to rats whose diet contained 40% of the dietary energy from fat and no differences in tumour development were noted between beef fat (low in PUFA), lard (moderate amount of PUFA) or corn oil (high in PUFA) as the fat sources. However, on repeating the experiment with only 5% of the dietary energy from fat, corn oil showed the highest development of tumours of the three fats. Critics say that the latter diet would have been the only one of the three at that level of fat to contain enough essential fatty acids and therefore the experimental conditions were not comparable.

Epidemiological data also do not point to diets high in PUFA having any extra risk of colo-rectal cancer. Thus, in those countries with higher saturated fat intakes (low PUFA intakes) there is a higher rate of colo-rectal cancer than in countries were PUFA intake is higher. In the USA, where the PUFA content of the diet has increased, CHD has decreased and there is no evidence of any unfavourable disease pattern developing, but rather a substantial decline in death rates from all causes.

In 1981 the P/S ratio in the UK was considered too low at 0.23, but during the 1980s there was some indication that it was rising, although by the end of the decade the national diet was still far from the goal of 0.45. There is a body of opinion in the UK which would be in favour of increasing the recommended P/S ratio beyond 0.45 to 1.0. Indeed, data from the Seven Countries Study indicated a further reduction of risk of CHD at higher ratios (see Fig. 7.14). If the intake of PUFA in the diet is increased, it is important that the levels of intake of vitamin E are also adequate (see discussion of antioxidant nutrients below).

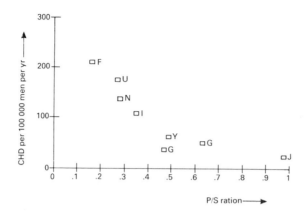

Fig. 7.14 — The relationship between P/S ratio and incidence of CHD in men aged 40–59 from the Seven Countries Study. Abbreviations as for Fig. 7.13. (Modified from Shaper, 1988.)

Starch and protein

Starch affects plasma VLDL by raising the triacylglycerols (TG) but has little effect on the cholesterol level. However, the effect is not sustained as the TG level drops again to its original level in a short period (days).

There is some evidence that animal protein (especially casein) may raise serum cholesterol level in comparison with plant proteins. This has been tentatively attributed to the amino acid pattern.

Dietary fibre

Communities that eat diets high in dietary fibre usually have a low mean plasma cholesterol level compared with those eating diets low in dietary fibre. However, there may be many other factors involved besides just the fibre content and it may be difficult to separate these. Although some isolated dietary fibres (e.g. pectin) have been shown to reduce raised cholesterol levels, others (e.g. cellulose) do not do so. Indeed, some foods high in dietary fibre have a marked effect on lowering raised cholesterol levels, while others do not. This is not unexpected, as dietary fibre from different sources is very different in composition. Under controlled conditions, plasma cholesterol levels of those on a western diet fall with diets high in oats (porridge) or legumes (Fig. 7.15). On the other hand, wheat fibre does not lower plasma cholesterol.

The possible mechanisms by which beans bring about this reduction in cholesterol level are given in Table 7.6. The effect is likely to be due to the high level of dietary fibre, but other factors such as the level of saponins have not yet been ruled out.

Alcohol

Generous intakes of alcohol may lead to hypertriglyceridaemia, but the plasma cholesterol level is not affected. However, moderate alcohol intakes can lead to raised

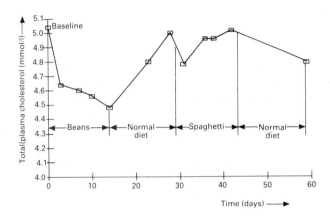

Fig. 7.15 — Change in cholesterol level of healthy young men during daily consumption of 450g of canned baked beans or spaghetti. (Modified from Shutler *et al.*, 1989.)

Table 7.6 — Possible mechanisms for hypocholesterolaemic effect of certain dietary fibres

---

- Increased fibre intake may be associated with decrease in fat and cholesterol intake, because foods high in fibre tend to be low in these components.

- Inhibition of absorption of dietary cholesterol — (e.g. by phytosterols in fibre-rich foods)

- Enhanced faecal excretion of cholesterol via bile owing to binding with fibre

- Enhanced faecal excretion of bile salts owing to binding with fibre

- Reduction in cholesterol synthesis by inhibition of rate limiting step — e.g. by short-chain fatty acids produced in the colon by fermentation of dietary fibre

---

HDL which may be advantageous in protecting from CHD. For further discussion of alcohol as a risk factor in CHD see Chapter 1.

Sucrose
This has no effect on blood cholesterol level and at the normal intake levels (20–25% of dietary energy — the amount normally present in British diets) it is not uniequivocally

established that it does have any specific triacylglycerol raising effect in normal people, despite the bad publicity against sugar!

Antioxidant nutrients

CHD is a multifactorial disease, meaning that many factors are involved in its aetiology, diet being only one. As far as diet is concerned, although most nutritionists agree that the fat content and type in the diet are important in the aetiology of CHD, it is unlikely to play a unique role in this respect. Even if fat is an important causative determinant of CHD, there is sufficient doubt as to its precise role to allow for other dietary factors to be involved.

Recently there has been interest in a possible protective role for antioxidant nutrients. The antioxidant nutrients are taken as the sum of a number of nutrients and pronutrients which are either directly antioxidant in nature, or are co-factors of enzymes involved in antioxidant activity in the body. These are:

vitamins A, C, E + β-carotene + selenium

Recent analyses of epidemiological evidence suggest that low levels of antioxidant nutrients, as assessed by their levels in the blood, are associated with increased risk of coronary heart disease. To study this further, two very large-scale intervention studies are currently underway in which groups of people are being given antioxidant nutrient supplements or placebo (they do not know which — i.e. it is a 'blind' trial) in large-scale trials to assess the efficacy of antioxident nutrient treatment on the incidence of CHD.

Working in concert, the antioxidant nutrients may reduce the effects of damaging oxidation reactions in the body, often initiated by highly reactive **free radicals**. These free radicals may be absorbed from the food (e.g. food that has been oxidized as a result of contact with oxygen in the atmosphere or severe processing) or may be made in the body. It is suggested that high levels of PUFA in the diet may lead to some peroxidation with free radical formation if the body is deficient in antioxidant nutrients. Under some circumstances, oxygen circulating in the body in the normal way (carried by haemoglobin) can form very reactive species such as singlet oxygen, which can be rendered harmless by antioxidants.

It has been suggested over recent years that the presence of high levels of free radicals and other reactive species within the body may promote the progression of certain degenerative diseases, including atherosclerosis and cancer. In atherosclerosis, which is of particular interest here, the presence of free radicals in the bloodstream particularly affects LDLs, which are most susceptible to oxidation, producing modified LDL. It has been shown that these modified LDL particles are not taken up by the cell LDL receptors (Fig. 7.8) in the normal way, but are engulfed by macrophages in the bloodstream. These macrophages become lipid-laden and attach themselves as 'foam cells' (Fig. 7.8) to the inside lining of arteries. The presence of foam cells is characteristic of atherosclerotic plaque.

Animal experimentation bears out the antioxidant hypothesis for the aetiology of CHD, as animals made deficient in antioxidant nutrients can be shown to develop damaging changes to arterial walls. Vitamin E has been shown to block the modification of LDL by oxidizing chemical species.

In addition to the effects of free radicals on LDL, it is also proposed that the presence of oxidized lipid inside the arterial plaque can lead to biochemical changes which result in a greater risk of thrombus formation.

Salt

Fruit and vegetables are naturally high in potassium and low in sodium, but nevertheless, most western diets are both high in sodium and low in potassium. This is because potassium in vegetables is leached out during cooking and poured away with water and sodium is added during cooking as salt. For the major part of human evolution, however, diets were more likely to have contained an abundance of potassium and a low level of sodium. Human beings seek the addition of salt to food because it acts as a flavour enhancer.

The relationship between salt intake and hypertension has been a subject for debate in medicine for some time. In healthy young adults the systolic blood pressure is about 120 mm Hg, and the diastolic pressure about 80. (When blood pressure is measured, two pressures are recorded: one when the left ventricle of the heart contracts — the systolic pressure; and the other when it relaxes — the diastolic pressure.) The diastolic pressure is more reliable than the systolic pressure, as it is less susceptible to physiological changes, e.g. those caused by exercise.

There is usually a gradual rise of blood pressure as age advances, and at about 65 years the mean figure in the western world is about 160/90. But the rise with age is variable. Mild hypertension occurs when diastolic pressure is 90—105, moderate hypertension when it is 105—120 and severe hypertension when it exceeds 120. However, increase in blood pressure with age is not inevitable: it does not occur in most animals or in some humans. In some primitive people there is no rise in blood pressure as age advances, e.g. in some of the people of the New Guinean Islands.

Japan has the highest incidence of strokes in the world and also the greatest incidence of high blood pressures. Indeed, the Japanese are some of the most avid salt eaters in the world. Their intake may be as high as 30 g per person per day — about twice that of the British. Although hypertension is commonly linked with obesity, it is possible for thin people to develop it.

No relationship was found between blood pressure and salt intake in the Framingham study (described above), but on the other hand, it is very difficult to accurately establish the habitual intake of salt of an individiual from one or two observations. Interpretation of data is difficult because of individual variation in response to salt. Even animal models show this. Thus, rats can be made to show hypertension on a high salt diet, but this will depend on the strain of the rat.

The first dietary guidelines to be published in the States (McGovern, 1977) recommended that the salt intake be reduced to about 3 g/person/day. This was criticised as being based on insufficient evidence. COMA (1984) recommended no increase in salt intake and that consideration should be given to decreasing it. Current attitudes tend to be that a 'blanket' recommendation on reducing salt intake would be of little value: it would not be of benefit to most people but only certain individuals, who should be given advice accordingly.

Summary of diet and CHD

Expected percentage changes in plasma cholesterol which might be achieved by changing dietary habits are shown in Fig. 7.16. As can be seen, it is predicted from this data that changing intake and type of dietary fat will have the greatest impact on plasma cholosterol. Little allowance is made in such predictions for other factors of more recent interest such as antioxidant nutrient status.

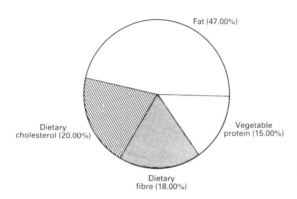

Fig. 7.16 — Expected percentage changes in plasma total cholesterol resulting from dietary modification. Modifications are: fat (from 40% energy of the diet as fat to 30%, with a change in the P/S ratio from 0.4 to 1.0); cholesterol (from 500 to 170 mg per day); dietary fibre (from 20 to 40 g per day); vegetable protein (from 30 to 50 g per day). (Data from Kay and Truswell, 1980.)

Soft water

In at least nine countries there has been found to be a significant negative association between the hardness of the drinking water and mortality from CHD. The harder the drinking water, the lower the death rate from CHD. Changes in the water supplied to a number of towns in the UK have also coincided with corresponding changes in the incidence of deaths from CHD — leading to further evidence that the suggestion of the association is not simply the results of chance.

No satisfactory explanation of this observation has yet been established. Soft water contains less calcium carbonate, magnesium and sulphate and more sodium than hard water. It has also been suggested that soft water is deficient in vanadium. Moreover, soft water picks up extra zinc, cadmium, iron, copper and lead from pipes. Hypotheses currently put forward are:

(a) Soft water has less vanadium. This mineral interferes with the synthesis of cholesterol and accelerates its breakdown and so can reduce the concentration of cholesterol in plasma.

(b) Cadmium — this is higher in soft water. It concentrates in the kidney and can induce hypertension in rats.

(c) Calcium — this is lower in soft water, the hardness of water being principally due to calcium content. There is some evidence that high blood pressure may be related to a low calcium intake. Of course, calcium in the water provides only part of totaldietary calcium and it would°be the total value which would be important. Working in the USA in the 1980s, McCarron (1984) studied the HANES 1 data (an enormous dietary survey of Americans) and found that hypertension was most significantly associated with low calcium intake of all the dietary variables. Interestingly, he found no link with sodium intake. Other studies also support the notion that low calcium intakes are associated with high blood pressure. But the exact mechanism by which calcium reduces blood pressure is not known. More work, especially more clinical studies are required before scientists can make general recommendations on calcium to the public.

Prevention and Treatment of CHD by Diet

Prevention
Stage I of atherosclerosis (Fig. 7.6) is the appropriate and desirable point to attack for the prevention of CHD. Prevention should begin in early childhood, with emphasis placed on the avoidance of hypercholesterolaemia. In the case of raised blood cholesterol levels, the use of drugs to reduce serum cholesterol level has often proved less promising than previously thought. It is particularly important that drugs used should be safe and have minimal side effects as they may be used for a considerable portion of a lifetime. Effective treatment by diet may be more acceptable in the longterm.

Normal serum lipids are those in which the cholesterol concentration of the blood is 4.7 mmol/l or less and fasting serum triacylglycerol levels are below 150 mg percent. Goals may not be achievable in all instances but, none them less, should be approached as basic objectives. For people with hyperlipidaemia due to diet, current recommendations are:

(a)   to restore weight to normal

(b)   to reduce saturated fat

(c)   to limit dietary cholesterol.

Other dietary modifications could be introduced, as outlined in this chapter, such as raising the intake of PUFAs and antioxidant nutrients to reduce atherosclerosis and supplementing the diet with calcium to reduce hypertension; but these measures do not have any official sanction at the moment, at least in the United Kingdom.

Dietary factors affecting HDL are different from those that act on LDL or plasma total cholesterol. Alcohol consumption produces a higher HDL level if taken in moderation, while obesity is associated with low HDL concentrations. Obesity and its relationship with disease is a subject of Chapter 6.

Intervention
Attempts to change diets in communities particularly at risk have been made in some parts of the world. The results of some recent multifactorial intervention trials are very

encouraging, for example, a primary prevention programme in N. Karelia (Finland) and a secondary prevention trial (i.e. among people who have survived a myocardial infarction) in Helsinki. However, there are not enough data from well-designed primary prevention trials worldwide. There may be many reasons for this, but they do require a lot of money, patience and persistence and medical scientists have to compete for relatively small short-term grants.

Regression of established atherosclerosis

It has been shown that severe atherosclerotic lesions (60% occlusion) can be experimentally induced in rhesus monkeys by feeding a high cholesterol, high fat diet. In these experiments, the effects were then reversed to give normal plasma cholesterol levels and only 26% luminal occlusion on cholesterol- and fat-free diets. However, great improvements of extensive calcified and fibrotic plaques in humans should not be expected, particularly as compliance to prescribed diets is often not good. Certainly humans would not tolerate the stringent diets fed to the monkeys.

Prevention of thrombosis is another approach to the prevention of CHD, which would be particularly relevant when there is already existing severe atherosclerosis. There is impressive evidence in rats that high linoleic acid in the diet will delay thrombosis. PUFAs found in fish oil and Eskimo diets also appear to diminish the tendency to thrombosis (see Chapter 5). Some other foods, such as onions and garlic, reduce platelet aggregation and therefore thrombotic tendency, but effects may be small.

CONCLUSION

Coronary heart disease continues to be one of the greatest causes of death in Britain. There is little evidence so far that the incidence is declining as rapidly as has happened in some other industrialized countries, notably the USA.

Epidemiological studies have identified a very wide range of possible risk factors for CHD, many of which are not diet related. All those studies analysed so far show three 'primary' risk factors for CHD: a high blood cholesterol level (hypercholesterolaemia), a high blood pressure (hypertension) and smoking. There is evidence that both the first two factors can be manipulated by diet.

Atherosclerosis is a fundamental condition to the development of CHD and human beings are very susceptible to it. In the lipid hypothesis for the formation of CHD it is proposed that a high level of saturated fat in the diet promotes a raised plasma cholesterol level, which encourages the deposition of cholesterol in the lining of the artery, forming plaque. Plaque can be mineralized and undergo other changes to proceed to complex lesions, whose surfaces may secrete biochemical messages which attract platelets from the blood, initiating thrombus formation. A heart attack happens suddenly, as a result of a thrombus becoming detached from the wall of the coronary artery, and travelling down in the blood stream to smaller arterial vessels (in the normal branching of the arterial system), until it reaches one which is narrow enough for the thrombus to become lodged. This event precludes further flow of blood along that part of the arterial system and the heart muscle becomes starved of oxygen.

Although the consensus opinion of nutritionists is that total dietary fat (and saturated fat in particular) plays a central role in the aetiology of CHD, and considerable evidence has accumulated to indicate this is so, this hypothesis is not proven and may never be. It is clear that more than a single dietary factor is involved in the development of CHD. For example, there is evidence that dietary fibre content of the diet and its type may be important, and recently interest has been shown in the protective role of the antioxidant nutrients. This has led to the organization of at least two large population intervention studies, the results of which will be available within the next few years. In the meantime, guidelines on eating for health have been published to encourage the public to change their eating habits. Dietary guidelines give recommendations based on 'the state of the art' and are likely to be refined as more information becomes available.

REFERENCES

COMA (1984) *Diet and cardiovascular disease*. Department of Health and Social Security. Health and Social Subjects No. 28. HMSO, London.

Connor, W. E. and Connor, S. J. (1972) The key role of nutritional factors in the prevention of coronary heart disease. *Preventative Medicine*. **1**, 49–83.

Duthie, G. G., Wahle, K. W. J. and James, W. P. T. (1989) Oxidants, antioxidants and cardiovascular disease. *Nutrition Research Reviews* **2**, 51–61.

Editorial (1984) Is reduction of blood cholesterol effective? *Lancet* i, 317–318.

Grundy, S. M. (1986) Cholesterol and coronary heart disease: a new era. *Journal of the American Medical Association*. **256** (20), 2849–2858.

Gurr, M. I., Borlack, N and Ganatra, S. (1989) Dietary fat and plasma lipids. *Nutrition Research Reviews* 2, 63–86.

Judd, P. A. and Truswell, A. S. (1985) Dietary fibre and blood lipids In: Leeds, A. R. (ed.) *Fibre perspectives* John Libbey, London.

Kay, R.M. and Truswell, A.S. (1980) Dietary fiber: effects on plasma and biliary lipids in man. In: Spiller, G.A. and Kay, R.M. (eds) *Medical aspects of dietary fiber*. Plenum Press, New York.

McCarron, D.A., Morris, C.D., Henry, H.J. and Stanton, J.L. (1984) Blood pressure and nutrient intakes in the United States. *Science*. **224**, 1392–1398.

McGovern, G. (1977) *Dietary goals for the United States*. Select Committee on Nutrition and Human Needs. Jan. 1977. Government Printing Office, Washington, D.C.

Padley, F. B. and Podmore, J. (eds) (1985) *The role of fats in human nutrition*. Ellis Horwood, Chichester, England.

Shaper, A. G. (1988) *Coronary heart disease: risks and reasons*. Current Medical Literature Ltd, London.

Shutler, S. M., Bircher, G. M., Tredger, J. A., Morgan, L. M., Walker, A. F. and Low, A. G. (1989) The effect of daily baked bean *(Phaseolus vulgaris)* consumption on the plasma lipid levels of young, normo-cholesterolaemic men. *British Journal of Nutrition* **61**, 257–265.

Vergroesen, A. J. and Crawford, M. (1989) *The role of fats in human nutrition*. 2nd edition. Academic Press, London.

8

Diabetes and diabetic diets
Anthony Leeds

Introduction
This chapter deals with the ways in which attitudes to diabetes and its management has changed over the years. It concentrates in particular on dietary management. Over the last 15 years or so, a number of exciting new developments have taken place in our understanding of the relation between diet and diabetes. However, before commencing on a discussion of this, it is necessary to discuss briefly the background to the disease.

BLOOD GLUCOSE REGULATION
The normal fasting level of blood glucose is about 4.4–5.6 mmol/l (80–100 mg/100 ml blood). After eating a meal containing carbohydrate, the level rises temporarily to 6.7–7.8 mmol/l. After fasting for 24 h or more, the blood glucose level is maintained at 3.3–3.9 mmol/l. Even with a very low intake of carbohydrate, the blood glucose level does not normally fall below 3.3 mmol/l. A low level of glucose in the blood is called **hypoglycaemia** and is as harmful to the brain as is lack of oxygen. A high level of glucose in the blood is called **hyperglycaemia** and, if greater than about 10 mmol/l, can lead to glucose in the urine (called **glycosuria**).

Factors which Regulate Blood Glucose
The blood glucose level at any point in time is a consequence of the rate at which glucose is entering and leaving the blood stream. Available carbohydrates in the diet tend to raise the level, but some of this is stored as **glycogen** in the liver, for release as and when it is required. This action of the liver in helping to maintain a constant level of blood glucose is called the **glucostat** function of the liver.

The glucostat function of the liver
The liver is the key organ in regulating blood glucose. When the blood glucose is high, the liver takes up glucose and stores it as glycogen. When the blood glucose is low, there

is net loss of glucose from the liver to the blood stream, by the breakdown of glycogen to glucose (**glycogenolysis**). Another way the liver can increase the output of glucose into the blood is by converting amino acids, lactate from muscle, or glycerol from split triacylglycerols in adipose tissue to glucose by a process known as **gluconeogenesis,** In addition to the liver controlling blood glucose level, there is also control from several **hormones**. The factors which tend to raise or lower blood glucose level are shown in the Table 8.1.

Table 8.1— Factors which tend to lower or raise blood glucose level

Lower	Raise
Fasting	Eating
Glycosuria (in diabetics)	Glycogenolysis *action of*: adrenalin
Insulin	glucagon
Physical activity	Gluconeogenesis
	Insulin antagonists growth hormone cortisol

Hormonal factors tending to lower blood glucose
The most important factor tending to lower blood glucose is the **insulin** secreted by the beta cells of the pancreatic islets of Langerhans. This lowers blood glucose in several ways, but the main one is by promoting the transport of glucose into the cells (without insulin, glucose cannot pass into the cells). Inside the cell the glucose can be oxidized, deposited as glycogen or converted to fat or amino acids, and insulin activates key enzymes in all of these pathways.

Hormonal factors tending to raise blood glucose
Glycogenolysis (which tends to raise blood glucose) is promoted by two hormones: **adrenalin** and **glucagon**. Adrenalin is released by the adrenal glands in response to stress, and glucagon is secreted by the alpha cells of the pancreatic islets of Langerhans. Both of these cause glycogen breakdown by activating the enzyme phosphorylase. In long-term starvation gluconeogenesis is a more important source of glucose than glycogenolysis, as the supplies of glycogen in the liver rapidly reduce. Under conditions of starvation it is normal for much gluconeogenesis to be provided by the breakdown of fat reserves. This releases fatty acids, which, together with their breakdown products the **ketone bodies** can be utilized by most tissues for energy. Glucagon, adrenalin and cortisol promote gluconeogenesis in different ways as follows:

Glucagon: stimulates enzymic pathways from amino acids to glucose
Adrenalin: inhibits the secretion of insulin
Cortisol: stimulates synthesis of enzymes responsible for gluconeogenesis.

Thus these hormones act in concert to increase blood glucose level partly by increasing glucose inflow into the blood and partly by reducing its outflow into the tissues.

DIABETES MELLITUS

Diabetes is a disease characterized by a high blood sugar and a relative or absolute lack of insulin. This may be associated with an excretion of glucose in the urine in the untreated state. It is usually caused by an insufficient secretion of insulin by the pancreas. At the same time there may be an excess of glucagon, which therefore raises the blood glucose level. Although the blood glucose level is high, the glucose cannot enter the cells because of the lack of insulin and, therefore, the untreated diabetic shifts from carbohydrate metabolism to fat metabolism for energy, which results in the formation of ketone bodies and in severe cases can cause acidosis with the formation of acetone which can be detected on the breath.

The most commonly used test for diabetes is the **Glucose Tolerance Test**. To carry out this test, glucose is given orally after fasting, at a dose of 1 g per kilogram body weight. In the normal person the blood glucose level rises from about 5 mmol/l to 7.8 mmol/l and then falls to normal within about 3 h. This fall comes from the release of insulin following the elevation of blood glucose. In the diabetic, the rise is much greater and will often greatly exceed 10 mmol/l, at which level glucose normally appears in the urine (i.e. the **renal threshold**). The fall is much slower than in normal people, and even the resting value may be as high as 16.7 mmol/l in some diabetics.

There are two main types of diabetes mellitus: **Type I** is also called the **juvenile type** because the age of presentation is in childhood. Injections of insulin in muscle tissue are needed for this type, so it is also called **Insulin-Dependent Diabetes Mellitus (IDDM)**. **Type II** is also called the **Maturity-Onset Diabetes (MOD)** or **Non-Insulin Dependent Diabetes Mellitus (NIDDM)** as the patient may not require injections of insulin for most of the course of the disease. MOD presents later in life.

There are differences in age of onset between the two types: IDDM peaks at 4–5 yrs and 11 yrs [juvenile diabetes can present later in life, around 25 or 30 years, but this is infrequent] and is thought to be related to difference in the way that individuals react to viral disease. It is likely to be common viruses which affect everybody which are at the root of the problem. These viruses grow in glandular tissue like the pancreas and can cause the problems under some conditions, even though normally they do not cause any lasting damage in most people. It is thought that in certain individuals an abnormal reaction leads to damage in the beta cells of the islets of Langerhans, which produce insulin.

As a consequence of that abnormal response to the infection (which may be genetically determined, as diabetes is known to run in families), these people are unable to produce sufficient insulin in meet the metabolic requirements. The need for insulin is fundamental, as insulin is required to transport glucose across the cell membrane and into the cell, as well as influencing other enzyme mediated reactions in the body. Therefore, when levels of insulin are reduced, it is a serious situation and the child becomes very ill. The main effects are high blood glucose, glucose in the urine and large quantities of urine (osmotic diuresis occurs, as the presence of glucose in the urine attracts water to it by osmosis), so the patient becomes very thirsty. At the same time, fat and protein is being broken down in much greater amounts than normal and there is weight loss. A number of other changes are related to water and electrolyte balance, resulting in the child becoming very unwell. This will often be noticed as abnormal behaviour such as inability to do the usual things at school. Infections can also be present.

Treatment of the juvenile type is with exogenous insulin which is injected subcutaneously twice per day usually — in order to match the way the pancreas would normally produce insulin. Even with insulin injections, dietary management is also required. One of the problems in juvenile diabetes is to meet needs for growth but to restrict energy so that the blood glucose level does not get too high. At the turn of the century, energy restriction was much tighter for diabetics as insulin was not available. Children on these regimes did not grow normally, as they matured before they achieved their optimum height. This does not happen now.

Mature-onset diabetes usually presents over the age of 45 and may have some of the features already described, but, more characteristically, it presents with some of the complications of diabetes, such as coronary heart disease or infections. 70% of these patients are overweight or obese. These people have a relative lack of insulin rather than an absolute lack: there is enough insulin, but the way the peripheral tissue responds (the sensitivity) to insulin changes. For reasons which are not completely understood, the amount of insulin needed to produce a given effect increases. So the pancreas produces more insulin to match that requirement. Even patients who are obese, but not diabetic, show insulin insensitivity, which may be related to changes taking place in the cell membrane or in the conformation of the insulin receptor.

Whatever the mechanism, there is no doubt that in MOD there is insulin insensitivity and, as a consequence, the beta cells of the islets of Langerhans produce more insulin early on in the disease and this can be measured as a higher blood insulin level than normal. This compensatory mechanism operating in the early stages of the illness begins to fail as the years go by and the pancreas fails to keep up with the high insulin requirements. This is the stage at which MOD patients show diabetes.

After presentation, all that may be required early on in the disease is to encourage the patient to reduce weight by restricting energy intake. This will lead to changes in flux in the metabolic pathways, and an increase in insulin sensitivity of the tissues. Under such circumstances, the insulin that is produced from the pancreas may then be sufficient. If diet alone is not sufficient, then the second stage is to give diet therapy plus an oral hypoglycaemic agent.

The oral hypoglycaemic agents were discovered during World War II as a result of the investigations into new antibiotics, particularly the sulphonamides. One of these was accidentally found to lower blood glucose. That particular compound gave rise to a whole family of drugs which are now used for lowering blood glucose, and act by one or more of the following mechanisms:

(a)   stimulating the beta cells to produce more insulin;
(b)   acting on the peripheral tissue to potential the action of insulin;
(c)   modifying or slowing down the rate of absorption of glucose.

Normally for MOD patients, the combination of diet and oral glycaemic agents gives good control of blood glucose level. However, the response does depend on patient compliance with the therapy. There are some patients who will not do anything which the doctor suggests to them and others who follow the therapy instructions implicitly. Obviously, as the successful outcome of the treatment depends on good patient compliance, the majority of patients will do fairly well. When MOD patients have had the condition for, say, 25 years, the pancreatic tissue, as all tissues of the body, ages and aging tissue is unable to synthesize protein at the rate that it was able to do when it was younger. So there comes a time (65 or 70 years old) when even with maximum doses of oral hypoglycaemic agents plus diet, the pancreas is unable to synthesize enough insulin to meet the requirement. For these patients, exgenous insulin by injection may then be required, but only in small doses (in contrast to juvenile diabetes).

THE MANAGEMENT OF THE DISEASE

There are basically two problems in management — the management of the acute presentation and long-term management:

Acute presentation   This occurs in juvenile-type diabetes and is a very serious condition. The patient is usually an adolescent and he or she may be treated with electrolytes and insulin given intravenously and then transferred to twice-daily intramuscular insulin. It is important to carefully monitor recovery of body weight and normal growth. Some patients with juvenile diabetes may not be so severely ill at the time of presentation and the handling can be taken in a more relaxed way.

Long-term management   This involves day-to-day management of patients with a severe metabolic problem. These days, as we are able to monitor blood glucose, it is possible to directly measure the effects of treatment directly. Biochemical measurements have only been possible since the development of biochemistry in the later part of the 19th century. Before that, practitioners would look at the urine, and check for colour, taste and clarity. Taste was used quite often until the later part of the 19th century.

A sweet-tasting urine is typical of uncontrolled diabetes mellitus and should not be confused with diabetes insipidus. The term 'diabetes' refers to flow through the body and implies large quantities of urine, and 'mellitus' refers to the sweet taste. Diabetes insipidus is a totally different disease condition from diabetes mellitus, and is related to a disturbance in the secretion of an anti-diuretic hormone which results in the patient passing vast amounts of tasteless urine.

Of course, these days, actual tasting is not used. From the end of the last century we could actually measure reducing sugars in urine and then, with the development of enzymic chemistry in the late 1920s and early 1930s, we have been able to measure glucose in blood samples. Recently, dipsticks have been developed, which contain, in a small pack at the end of a stick, all the enzymes necessary for the detection of glucose. The pack contains filtration material, which holds back the red blood cells, and allows the serum to filter through to the enzyme and other reagents, and a colour develops in response to the amount of glucose in the blood. This colour can then be compared to a colour chart, or the dipstick pack can be placed in a refractometer, which will give a digital readout of the glucose level in two minutes. In this way it is now possible for patients to measure their own blood glucose. All it requires is for the patient to take a finger prick of blood. This is a tremendous advance in the management of diabetes, because, in the past, blood glucose control was very difficult because there was no useful means of monitoring progress.

The blood glucose level in a normal person is about 5 mmol/l (90 mg/dl) when fasting. In an uncontrolled diabetic it could be from 8 — 25 mmol per l and though the renal threshold for glucose varies, it might be between 13—15 mmol/litre, which is why the glucose spills over into the urine. In the past, when all we could do was to look at the glucose in the urine, one of the problems was the risk of overtreating and getting the blood glucose too low. If this happens, then the patient suffers from hypoglycaemia, feeling shaky, sweaty and light-headed; then the brain will not function and person passes out. If glucose becomes very low it is incompatible with life and for this reason, an overdose of insulin is fatal. In the past, there was a real danger of this happening, so it was common practice to aim for the blood glucose of diabetics to be kept close to the renal threshold. This was to facilitate monitoring of glucose in the blood: sometimes there was glucose in the urine, sometimes not. However, under this regime, the glucose level in the blood was about 13–15 mmol/l: much higher than normal.

We now know from some prospective studies done in Europe over the last 10 years, that the risk of complications of diabetes does relate to the excellence of glucose control. These investigations have involved up to 1000 diabetics who were divided into three groups:, *a well controlled group*, (which has no urine glucose and low blood glucose), a *middle group* (with middle values, less well controlled) and a third group, *the badly controlled group* (with glucose in the urine and high blood glucose). Analysis of data has shown that the last two groups are more likely to develop complications, particularly those affecting small blood vessels.

We now know that what we wish to achieve is a fasting level of blood glucose around 5 mmol/l and excursions of no more than 3 mmol/l after meals. It is clear that what we were doing before was not the best possible treatment. Now it is possible to change this and keep glucose levels very nearly normal, with the patients measuring their own blood glucose levels up to five times a day to make sure they do not go too low. They can balance dietary intake and exercise; they know how much to feed themselves in anticipation of major excercise.

Historical development of dietary management of diabetes
Although classification of the disease has changed over the centuries, we can be fairly confident that diabetes mellitus has been with mankind at least 3500 years. Indeed, there is mention of it in writing on an Egypian papyrus dating from about 1500 BC, in which a condition is described in which there is a great quantity of urine passed. The condition was treated by a diet which included dried fruit and honey. One thousand years later some Sanskrit manuscripts describe a disease in which the urine attracts insects — an observation compatible with the presence of glucose in the urine. Diabetes mellitus was also known to Greek physicians. However, there were not many records of diabetes between 150 AD and about the 17th century.

200 years ago, Matthew Dobson working in Liverpool was treating patients who had sugar in the urine, with more sugar in the diet — he reasoned that if sugar were lost, then it would need to be replaced. In the 17th century, Thomas Willis (Plate 8.1) described diabetes as characterized by sweet urine. He also indicated that he had a treatment for it

based on dietary intake restriction, although there are not enough records to know if his treatment really worked.

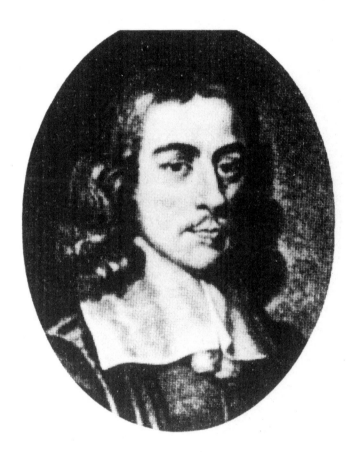

Plate 8.1 — Thomas Willis, Physician.

By the 19th century, dietary restriction was well recognized as beneficial for the condition. It is necessary to be careful in interpreting older records of diabetes, as we now recognize two types and in the older literature there is no such distinction. It is highly probable that those with the juvenile type did not survive very long, so that described in the old literature was probably for the maturity-onset type. In 1871, in the siege of Paris, when the Prussian army was outside Paris, preventing the movement of food into the city, starvation occurred. Some physicians noted that the condition of their diabetic patients improved — that dietary restriction had been beneficial, especially restriction of carbohydrate. As a consequence, carbohydrate restriction began to be used in the routine treatment of this condition. In the case of MOD, this was often treated by imposing diet restriction and then adding food back to the diet in increasing amounts, until there was sugar in the urine again. This level of intake was then regarded as the amount of energy that these patients should aim to consume.

Plate 8.2 shows the front page of a book written in 1779 by John Rollo, who was Surgeon-General to the Royal Artillery. He had an idea that diabetes was a disease of the stomach and that it was necessary to give the stomach a rest by prescribing this diet, which you see (Table 8.2) was one in which he suggested plain blood pudding and rancid old meats, adding up to a high fat intake. It is not known if the patients actually consumed this diet: often, compliance with prescribed diets is not good. Neither do we know the success rate for the diet.

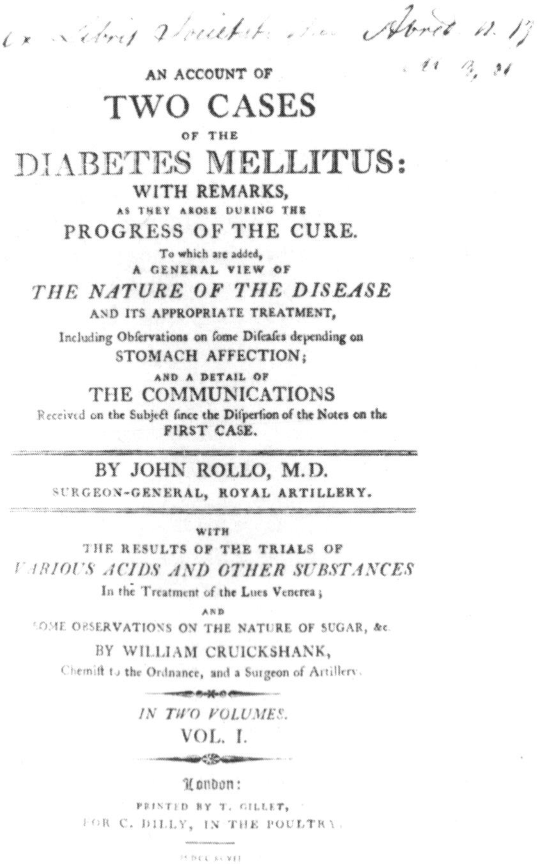

AN ACCOUNT OF

TWO CASES

OF THE

DIABETES MELLITUS:

WITH REMARKS,

AS THEY AROSE DURING THE

PROGRESS OF THE CURE.

To which are added,

A GENERAL VIEW OF

THE NATURE OF THE DISEASE

AND ITS APPROPRIATE TREATMENT,

Including Obfervations on fome Difeafes depending on

STOMACH AFFECTION;

AND A DETAIL OF

THE COMMUNICATIONS

Received on the Subjeĉt fince the Difperfion of the Notes on the

FIRST CASE.

BY JOHN ROLLO, M.D.

SURGEON-GENERAL, ROYAL ARTILLERY.

WITH

THE RESULTS OF THE TRIALS OF

VARIOUS ACIDS AND OTHER SUBSTANCES

In the Treatment of the Lues Venerea;

AND

SOME OBSERVATIONS ON THE NATURE OF SUGAR, &c.

BY WILLIAM CRUICKSHANK,

Chemift to the Ordnance, and a Surgeon of Artillery.

IN TWO VOLUMES.

VOL. I.

London:

PRINTED BY T. GILLET,

FOR C. DILLY, IN THE POULTRY.

Plate 8.2 — Front page of a book written in 1779 by John Rollo, in which he described diabetes as a disease of the stomach and prescribed a high fat diet containing 'rancid old meats' as dietary treatment.

Table 8.2 — John Rollo's diet for Captain David Meredith: 1797

Breakfast	1 $^1/_2$ pints of milk and $^1/_2$ pint of lime water mixed together; Bread and butter
Noon	Plain blood pudding — blood and suet only
Dinner	Game or old meats Fat and rancid old meats 'as fat as the stomach may bear'
Supper	As breakfast

Source: Anderson, 1965.

From 1870 onwards other improvements as well as dietary restrictions were attempted. About that time there was a potato diet and a porridge diet (30 oz porridge per day). The latter (Table 8.3a) is particularly interesting, because the energy content is not very great — about 700 kcals per day, and also the dietary fibre is only about 14 g per day (calculated from Paul and Southgate, 1978) (Table 8.3b) compared with today's UK average intake of between 10 and 20 g per day. It is now recognized that most adult men require about 3000 kcals and adult women around 2200 kcal per day. In addition, we now draw a distinction between water- soluble and insoluble dietary fibre. Soluble fibre has particular effects in the gut, and, as we shall see later, it is quite possible that the porridge diet did have beneficial effects on glucose absorption. Indeed, over the last 10 years in the USA, Dr Jim Anderson, a well-known researcher in this field, has been promoting porridge and high oat diets for his diabetic patients with considerable success.

Table 8.3a — The Porridge Diet

Breakfast	10 oz porridge with 1$^1/_2$ oz milk 1 egg
Lunch	1 oz brandy and 1 egg 10 oz porridge with lemon juice 6 oz cabbage with $^1/_8$ butter
Dinner	1 egg 10 oz porridge with $^1/_4$ oz grated Parmesan cheese 3$^1/_2$ oz French beans and $^1/_8$ oz butter

Source: Cammidge, 1920.

Table 8.3b — Analysis of Porridge Diet using *McCance and Widdowson's The Composition of Foods*

Percentage total energy as			Total energy (kcal)	Dietary fibre (g)
Carbohydrate	Protein	Fat		
43	18	39	715	14

Source: Paul and Southgate, 1978.

About a century ago, a typical dietary regime for the management of diabetes would contain only 11% of energy from carbohydrate; 12% would be from protein and 78% from fat. 192 g of fat per day is a very high intake of fat, which again raises the question of whether compliance was good. Fast days were also advocated in the latter part of the 19th century, so physicians gave their patients bran biscuits containing agar to deal with the constipation that ensued. We now know that both bran and agar would contain a lot of dietary fibre, which would not only have relieved the constipation, but would also have had beneficial effects on the gut in delaying glucose absorption.

Table 8.4 summarizes the historical development of dietary management of diabetes and brings us to the present day. Over the last 15 years there have been very marked changes in attitudes towards diabetic management. Now, energy intake is still controlled, but instead of a high fat, low carbohydrate diet, a low fat, high carbohydrate, high fibre diet is now advocated.

Table 8.4 — Summary of historical development of dietary management of diabetes

Replacement of lost sugars
Rest for the stomach
Energy restriction, including fast days
Carbohydrate restriction
High carbohydrate, high fibre

For the future, many new possibilities are in prospect to ease diabetic management. While results of research will continue to refine the dietary approach, it is more than possible that pancreatic islet cell transplantation will be introduced and diabetics will no longer need to inject themselves with insulin. Research along these lines is active at the moment and it is likely that the new approaches will be possible in 10 – 15 years time.

LATE COMPLICATIONS OF DIABETES

At the moment, then, diabetes cannot be cured, but a cure may not be a long way off as transplantation becomes successful. Transplantation technology is very advanced now, and it is likely that in 20 years time juvenile diabetics will be transplanted and most will do very well. In the meantime, we have to deal with the late complications of the disease. These effects largely involve blood vessels, although there are some other effects, like cataract formation, which develops in some patients. Cataract formation can be treated by surgery and replacement of the lens with an artificial lens.

Macrovascular complications

The main problems in diabetes are the macrovascular changes which are related to atherosclerosis. All human beings develop atherosclerosis; the critical thing is the rate at which it develops. In some people it never presents a problem throughout a long lifetime. However, in general, the older a person is, the more atherosclerosis is likely to be present. As a general rule, when 60% of the coronary arteries are covered by atherosclerotic plaque, a person is at high risk of developing some acute manifestation like a heart attack (**coronary heart disease** — CHD) or **peripheral vascular disease** (insufficient blood supply to the legs etc).

In diabetics the rate at which atherosclerosis develops is faster than in people who do not have diabetes. (There are other risk factors — the rate is also faster if you smoke, have high blood pressure or high blood cholesterol level.) All of those things together increase considerably the chances of getting atherosclerosis at a very young age.

Atherosclerosis is a multifactorial disease (see Chapter 7), but in diabetes some of the metabolic problems result in an acceleration of the atherosclerotic process. For example, excess insulin (which may happen on a chronic basis if diabetic control is not precise) encourages atherosclerosis formation. Traditional high fat, low carbohydrate diets prescribed 15 years ago are now known to be associated with high blood cholesterol levels and will increase the rate of formation of atherosclerosis. High incidences of CHD and peripheral vascular disease are found in diabetic patients in the age range 60–70 years, in whom an element of the disease complications is caused by the dietary managment as well as by the disease condition itself.

Expressing the normal mortality rate of non-diabetic individuals as 1, data for 1970 (Table 8.5) shows that young male diabetics are nine times more likely to die of CHD than are normal people at that age (although the absolute numbers are very low). In the older age groups where the absolute numbers rise, the relative mortality drops to between 2–4 x normal rates. Although there are no more recent figures than these, it is likely that the next published values will be lower than this as a result of better control of blood glucose levels in recent years.

Table 8.5 — Relative mortality from heart disease in diabetics

Age group	Mortality Rate	
(years)	Men	Women
25–35	9	7
35–44	4	7
45–54	2	4

Normal mortality rate of non-diabetic individuals =1.
Source: Bierman and Brunzell, 1978.

Microvascular complications

The microvascular complications are problems which develop in small blood vessels as a consequence of the effect of a high blood glucose level modifying protein structure and function — particularly those proteins of the small blood vessels. As a consequence the vessels may fail to allow the blood to flow freely through them — resulting in localized ischaemia. In addition, the vessels may leak and serum seep out into the surrounding tissue. All small blood vessels are affected, but there are three systems which are affected more severely than others:

The retina of the eye: Changes in the function of small blood vessels in the retina can lead to **retinopathy**, the consequence of this being that visual acuity may be reduced — so the person cannot see so clearly. These days, treatment can be given to slow down the rate of degeneration. In addition, the tighter control over blood glucose levels available over in the last 10 years or so will also prevent progression. The magnitude of the problem of retinal changes in diabetes is clear when it is realized that 1 in 5 people registered blind are blind as a consequence of diabetes. In the future this will not be the case.

The kidneys: Small blood vessels which supply the tubules of the kidney are also affected by the same process and **nephropathy** can result. The arterioles cease to function and then die, and some of the nephrons may also become necrotic. Gradually, with considerable loss of nephrons, renal function declines. One of the causes of death in (generally) older diabetics, is renal failure.

The nerves: Nerves affected are mainly along the long nerves to limbs. These are supplied with small blood vessels which enter the nerve sheath as the nerve travels down the limb. These blood vessels may also block off as described above and the nerve become ischaemic (blood supply is cut off). This leads to lack of oxygen and nutrient supply, which results in loss of function of long nerves. The condition is called **neuropathy**. Initially this shows as loss of fine sensory qualities such as the sensations of vibration, joint position and the ability to distinguish between different temperatures. Then, gradually, there may be a loss of motor function and then loss of all function. The autonomic nervous system can also be affected, so some patients lose motility in the gut and bladder. The duration of the diabetes will make a difference to the involvement of the nerves in this way, but so will the excellence of blood glucose control.

The tighter the control on blood glucose levels, the less likely diabetics are to develop microvascular changes, so now a great deal of effort is made to keep levels of glucose as normal as possible.

DIET IN LONG-TERM MANAGEMENT

There are four main considerations in undertaking long-term management of diabetes:

(a)   the excellence of diabetic control;
(b)   the vascular disease risk;

(c) the risk of hyperlipidaemia;
(d) avoiding an obese or overweight condition — it is best to aim for ideal body weight
     (see Chapter 6), as metabolic control will be better.

Similarly, in prescribing a diet the following variables need to be manipulated in diabetic diets:

> Dietary energy
> Sources of energy — especially fat or carbohydrate
> Dietary fibre
> Simple sugars.

In future, there may be other dietary variables, such as the choice of a high **chromium** intake. Chromium has been called a **glucose tolerance factor** as it helps to reduce levels of insulin required to effect blood glucose control. Barley grown on certain soils is particularly rich in chromium.

Most medical practitioners are agreed that energy in the diet should be controlled: unlimited amounts of energy lead to very poor blood glucose control. As far as the sources of energy in the diet are concerned, it was clear at the end of the 19th century that carbohydrate restriction could be beneficial for diabetics. However, in the 1930s, Himsworth showed that under some circumstances allowing a freer use of carbohydrate would still give just as good metabolic control. What he did not realize was that the type of carbohydrate used in the diabetic diet was important and that the processing of the starch can affect its digestion. It is now evident that the structure of the food is important, for example, whether or not it has been milled or cooked. The effect of food particle size can be seen commonly by the presence of entire, undigested maize (corn) kernels in the faeces, whereas cornflour is well digested.

If the diabetic diet is changed from the traditional low carbohydrate/high fat one to one high in carbohydrate and low in fat, by changing one energy source for another, this will have other compositional implications for the diet. This is because the starchy foods eaten will also be higher in dietary fibre. Therefore, in experimental situations designed to determine the effects of exchanging carbohydrate for fat as an energy source, it is not easy to separate the effects of fibre and the effect of carbohydrate.

Only a few reports are published in which reasonable attempts have been made to separate these effects. One experiment, conducted in Italy on 4 IDDM and 4 NIDDM patients, compared three different diets (Rivellese *et al.*, 1980):

(a) 53% of carbohydrate, 16 g fibre (usual Italian diet);
(b) 53% carbohydrate, 54 g fibre (Italian diet, with fibre-rich foods);
(c) 42 % carbohydrate and 20 g fibre (traditional low-carbohydrate diabetic diet);

(NB: As this study was carried out in Italy, this makes a difference as to the approach to treatment, which may vary from that in the UK. In some countries practitioners are much more liberal with insulin and a large number of MOD patients are on insulin injections, whereas in the UK those MOD diabetics prescribed injections are very few.)

In this experiment, glucose levels were significantly lower after the high-fibre diet (b), compared with either the traditional low-carbohydrate diabetic diet (c), or the usual

Italian diet (a). Despite a substantial difference in carbohydrate content, the two low-fibre diets (a and c) gave similar blood glucose control.

Fig. 8.1 is taken from another clinical trial. This is the work of Dr Jim Anderson in the USA (Anderson and Ward, 1979). He studied eight insulin-dependent diabetics over 20 days. He used a standard control diet with 43% of energy from carbohydrate, in a 'run in' period, when fasting blood glucose levels were high (about 8.0 mmol/l). After treatment with a high fibre diet (70 g dietary fibre per day), the insulin doses required began to fall, and there was also a fall in blood glucose levels (both fasting and postprandial (after a meal)) — despite the reduction in insulin dose. This means MOD patients treated with insulin could stop these injections and achieve the same or better metabolic control on a high fibre diet because insulin requirement has been reduced. Of course IDDM patients would still need to carry on with their injections, but the levels of insulin required could be reduced.

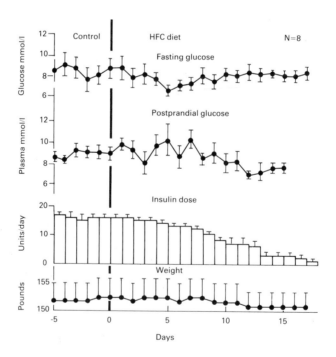

Figure 8.1 — Response of insulin-dependent diabetics to control diet (see text) and high fibre, high carbohydrate diet (HFC). From Anderson and Ward, 1979. Reproduced with permission from the American Journal of Clinical Nutrition.

It is now possible to measure precisely an individual's requirement for insulin by infusing glucose and insulin into the blood stream and determining exactly how much insulin is required to transfer glucose from the blood into peripheral tissues. These types of studies have shown quite clearly that high carbohydrate, high fibre diets do result in a reduction of the insulin requirement.

Effect on diabetic control of the source of dietary fibre
Most of the early studies of the effects of dietary fibre on diabetic control were carried out using wheat starches and wheat fibre. The aim of good diabetic control is to achieve a 24-hour blood glucose profile similar to that of a normal person, which would rise to a maximum level of 6.5 – 7.0 mmol/l to fall back promptly to around 5 mmol/l. High carbohydrate, high fibre diet using wheat bran, showed a tendency towards an improvement but was not very effective. To determine whether the *type* of dietary fibre made any difference, a study was carried out in Oxford to compare the traditional diabetic diet (40% energy as carbohydrate, 40% as fat and 15 g of fibre per day — designated the LC diet), with one high in carbohydrate and soluble fibre. The diet chosen for comparison was one containing a very high proportion of beans (designated HL — see Fig. 8.2). This comprised 61% carbohydrate, 18% fat, 21% protein and 96.6 g of fibre per day. This diet resulted in the whole of the glucose profile being lowered, with very marked changes in glucose levels. In the long term such a diet would have the effect of slowing down the metabolic processes which result in the microvascular changes.

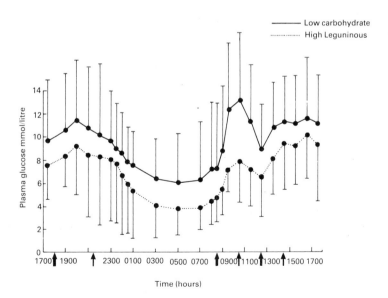

Figure 8.2 — Plasma glucose values, during 24 hours, of insulin-dependent diabetic patients on HL (high legume and cereal fibre diet) and LC (low carbohydrate, traditional, diabetic diet). From Simpson *et al.*, 1981. Reproduced with permission from The Lancet.

However, most patients would find it unacceptable to eat the high quantities of beans consumed in the experimental diets illustrated in Fig. 8.2 It is known from several studies that if patients are given an opportunity to select food, they prefer to eat white rice and refined cereals rather than whole cereals, and fruit juice rather than whole fruit and they are not very keen on beans. These findings are certainly true of older patients. Young diabetics are more flexible and will modify their diets to eat large quantities of beans and other sources of soluble dietary fibre.

Although getting patients to eat beans is not easy, it is possible that fibre can be extracted from them and cooked in crisp bread or ordinary bread. The development of a high soluble-fibre white bread was carried out in the Department of Food Science and Technology at the University of Reading by Dr Peter Ellis (Ellis *et al.*, 1981.), who managed to incorporate as much as 15% (dry weight) of guar gum in the recipe. Guar gum is extracted from the cluster bean and was chosen because it was commercially available and had been used for a long time in foodstuffs. This bread was used in experimental studies with diabetics and was shown to be very acceptable. The use of guar has now been extended into the development of biscuits and pasta products, which may be available commercially in the near future. These products have been shown to reduce the glucose and insulin levels in diabetics and also to reduce the plasma cholesterol level. In fact, the pharmaceutical industry has also risen to the challenge and has now produced guar granules, and other products for the same purpose.

Fig. 8.3 shows the effects on glucose and insulin levels of incorporating soluble fibre (guar gum and pectin) into a breakfast meal for eight non-insulin-requiring diabetics. In the upper panel you see the glucose responses, starting from an abnormally high value in these diabetic patients of about 8 mmols/l, and rising up above the renal threshold, above 15 mmol/l for the controls (no guar or pectin added to breakfast); whereas the lower dotted line is the breakfast test meal containing soluble fibre. In the bottom panel the insulin responses are given. On high soluble fibre, lower glucose levels were achieved with a lower insulin output. Thus demand on the pancreas was lower, despite the fact that the glucose levels were also lower.

Proposed mechanisms for the action of soluble fibre in reducing blood glucose levels
Soluble fibre may act in the gut in a number of different ways — it is not known which of them is the most important (Fig. 8.4). It may have an effect on gastric filling: fibre may slow down eating, or the amount eaten may be rather less. Gastric emptying may be slowed down: if fibre did slow gastric emptying then delivery to the small intestine would be slower and so would digestion. The rates of reaction of enzymes on substrates in the small intestine (rate of digestion) may be slower, and there is some evidence for that. The rate of absorption may be slower, because of the increased viscosity of the gut contents.

In addition to these possible changes, other functions may be changed. The motility, the pH and hormonal responses in the gut may be altered. The gut is the largest endocrine organ in the body and produces a variety of hormones which control many metabolic events. The pattern of release of those hormones may be different on a high-soluble fibre diet, and this may have important metabolic consequences.

The gut is also a dynamic organ which responds to stresses — for example, the gut grows during pregnancy. Another example is that the distal part of the gut will respond if

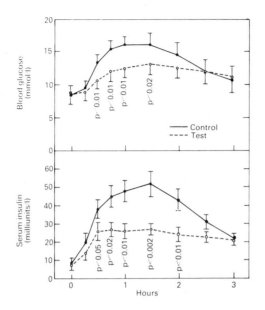

Fig. 8.3 — Blood glucose and serum insulin concentrations (mean ± SEM) in eight non-insulin-requiring diabetics after breakfast meals with (test) and without (control) pectin and guar gum. From Jenkins *et al.*, 1976. Reproduced with permission from The Lancet.

there is damage to the upper part, so that the lower portion of the small intestine will take over the role of the upper part of the gut. Fibre, especially soluble fibre, may delay the absorption of nutrients, so that they are absorbed further down the intestine. That would have the effect of slowing all the digestive responses, which might lead to overflow of food into the colon.

In most physiology text books the colon is described as a storage organ, which only absorbs water and electrolytes. These days, the colon is gradually revealing its secrets to those who are prepared to persist in the difficult task of investigating it. It is likely that in the next 10 years or so scientists may discover that it is a much more important organ than previously thought.

There is no doubt that much fermentation of food residues occurs in the human colon. In fact, the colon probably plays a similar role in man as the rumen plays in a ruminant. However, refined western diets do not allow much material to pass through into the organs, as most of it is digested and absorbed with little residue. Therefore, colon fermentation on such diets may be limited. This may not have been so for our ancestors during the course of evolution, who would have been eating a diet of very different composition with a much higher content of fibre. Then much more food would have passed into the colon and there would have been much more fermentation. Fermentation of soluble fibre in the colon leads to the formation of **short-chain fatty acids** (SCFA), which have considerable effects on a number of metabolic pathways, including the synthesis of cholesterol (see Chapter 7) in the liver. Therefore, it is likely that human

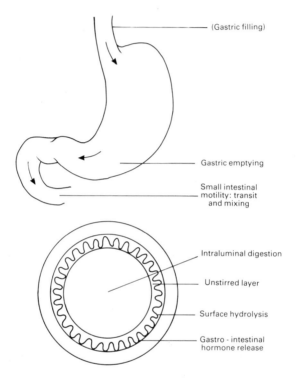

Fig. 8.4 — Factors affecting intestinal absorption which may be modified by dietary fibre. From Leeds, 1982.

metabolism would have been different under these circumstances and that patterns of disease would also have been totally different as well.

Fig. 8.5 shows some evidence of different gastrointestinal hormone responses to high fibre diets. The particular hormone in question in Fig. 8.5 is GIP — gastric inhibitory peptide, which is one of the hormones released from the upper gut in response to meals. Insulin is released in response to release of GIP, so a reduced secretion of GIP would result in a reduced insulin response. Fig. 8.5 shows a very big difference in the release of this hormone in response to a high guar gum meals, compared with control meals, in both normal and diabetic people.

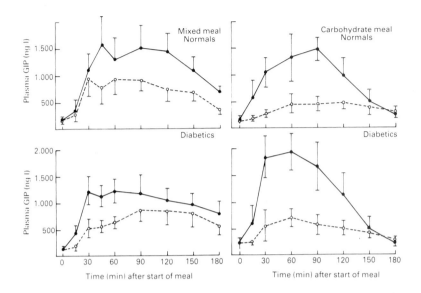

Fig. 8.5 —Effect of guar gum on the secretion of gastric inhibitory peptide (GIP) in normal and diabetic subjects after mixed and carbohydrate meals. ●—● = control meals (no guar gum); ○- - -○ = meals with 10g guar gum. From Morgan et al., 1979. Reproduced with permission.

Simple Sugars

In the 19th century, and even earlier, it began to be realized that diabetics had to avoid sugar in the diet, and this concept entered into traditional medical training. However, in recent years not only has the traditional low carbohydrate, high fat diet been challenged, but also the restrictive attitude to sugar. Recently, studies have been made of test meals given to diabetics, in which the amount of sugar have been varied. From the results it can be concluded that there is no need to worry too much about sugar as long as it is taken as part of a mixed meal with a high content of dietary fibre and complex carbohydrate (starch) to give the necessary slowing down of sugar absorption. So the advice now is that it is really not necessary to restrict sugar for diabetics, as long as the sugar is taken as part of a suitable meal. Sugar taken between meals has a very marked effect in raising blood glucose level and is not recommended.

In 1982 the British Diabetic Association (BDA) published recommendations for diets for diabetics and these are summarized in Table 8.6. Since that time considerable amounts of new data have been published and it is likely that the next recommendations will contain a number of important changes.

Although there are no recommendations about the *types* of starch, it is probable that the next set of recommendations will discuss the way in which different types of starches are digested at different rates. No specific recommendation was made about aiming for a high fibre diet in the 1980s recommendations, However, the American Diabetic

Table 8.6 — A summary of the main recommendations for diets for diabetics
for the 1980s

---

(1) Dietary energy in relation to energy requirement remains the most important
feature of diabetic management. It is important that it is balanced by a qualified
dietitian.

(2) Energy from carbohydrate need not be low carbohydrate (CHO) but should be
from polysaccharides (starches), especially with high dietary fibre. y higher fibre
Soluble

(3) Sugars should be excluded. — mixed meal provided
quantity not too great

(4) The diet should be characterized by low dietary fat. The energy from CHO
should be more than 50% of the total energy, and the energy fat should be no
more than 35%.

(5) Carbohydrate portions remain essential for those on insulin therapy.

(6) Obese diabetics can lose weight by any sound reducing diet.

(7) Diabetics should avoid excess sodium. *

(8) Alcohol is allowed, but the energy content should be taken into account.

(9) Speciality foods are of no particular value for diabetics. * not essential

---

Adapted from: British Diabetic Association, 1982.

Association has recently made some recommendations about the **amounts** of fibre in the
diet and it is likely that the BDA will make some specific recommendations soon. It is
likely that they will advocate higher fibre in the diet, and they may specify that it is
soluble fibre.

It is likely that the next set of recommendations will be less dogmatic about sugar
intake and that they will suggest that sugars as part of a mixed meal need not be of
particular concern, provided that the quantity is not too great. The advice on fat intake is
consistent with the recommendations for the general population as made in the COMA
(DHSS, 1984) Report on *Diet and cardiovascular disease*.

Suitable methods of weight reduction could include the patient joining Weight
Watchers or using Slimming Club magazines. However, faddist diets such as the
Beverley Hills diet are not recommended. (The Beverley Hills diet might comprise a
grapefruit on one day followed by a pineapple the next day, a lobster the next day etc.)
These diets are totally unbalanced and dangerous for diabetics.

As far as sodium is concerned, there is no suggestion that sodium in the diet interacts
with carbohydrate metabolism, but everyone should consider sodium in the diet in
relation to its epidemiological association with stomach cancer and hypertension (high
blood pressure). Despite the lack of strong evidence in the general population, relating

high levels of sodium in the diet to hypertension, it will certainly not do any harm to reduce the sodium in the diets of most people. Some people, who are very sensitive to sodium and who do get raised blood pressure for this reason, would benefit greatly by reducing their salt intakes.

Alcohol is allowed up to a point, but obviously no-one would want to see excessive drinking in diabetics anymore than in the normal population.

Although specialist diabetic foods, like jellies and squashes, might be useful for treats for children, who otherwise might feel deprived in comparison with their normal friends, there is no medical reason to advocate them.

In general, the BDA recommendations on diets for diabetics for the 1980s also apply largely to the general population and are consistent with the American and Canadian recommendations for diabetics which were produced for the 1980s. However, with the new set of guidelines now published in America, once more the USA is ahead of Britain in nutritional matters.

CONCLUSION

The last ten years have seen very considerable changes in the dietary regimes used with diabetics. The traditional diabetic diet was one high in fat and low in carbohydrate. Evidence is accumulating that such a diet may be inferior in terms of control of blood glucose level to one high in carbohydrate and dietary fibre, for both insulin-dependent (Type I) and non-insulin dependent diabetics (Type II). In addition, the high fat content of the traditional diet may lead to long-term health implications, particularly in terms of increased risk of coronary heart disease.

As a consequence of the results of scientific investigation on the metabolic consequences of high versus low carbohydrate diets, with the presence or not of fibre (especially soluble fibre), major diabetic organizations worldwide have now published guidelines on diet for diabetics, which are broadly in line with those currently advocated for the general public for limiting the risks of macrovascular disease. The diabetic is now encouraged to eat wholegrain cereals, plenty of fruit and vegetables and beans, and to avoid too much fatty food.

REFERENCES

Anderson, F. J. (1965) *Journal of the History of Medicine*, **20**, 163–164.
Anderson, J. W. and Ward, K. (1979) High carbohydrate, high fiber diets for insulin-treated men with diabetes mellitus. *American Journal of Clinical Nutrition.* **32**, 2312.
Birch, G. G. and Parker, K. J. (eds) (1983) *Dietary fibre*. Applied Science Publishers, London.
British Diabetic Association (1982) Dietary recommendations for diabetics for the 1980's — a policy statement by the British Diabetic Association. *Human Nutrition: Applied Nutrition,* **36A**, 378–394.
Cammidge, P. J. (1920) *Diabetic dieting and cookery*. ULP, London.
DHSS (1984) *Diet and cardiovascular disease*. The 'COMA Report'. Report on Health and Social Subjects No.28. HMSO, London.
Dreher, M. L. (1987) *Handbook of dietary fiber: an applied approach*. Marcel Dekker, New York.

Ellis, P.R., Apling, E.C., Leeds, A.R. and Bolster, N.R. (1981) Guar bread: acceptability and efficacy combined. Studies on blood glucose, serum insulin and satiety in normal subjects. *British Journal of Nutrition.* **46**, 267–276.

Jenkins, D. J. A., Leeds, A. R., Gassull, M. A., Wolever, T. M. S., Goff, D. V., Alberti, K. G. M. M. and Hockaday, T. D. R. (1976) Unabsorbable carbohydrates and diabetes: decreased post-prandial hyperglycaemia. *The Lancet ii*, 172–174.

Leeds, A. R. (1982) Modification of intestinal absorption by dietary fiber and fiber components. In: Vahouny, G. V. and Kritchevsky, D. (eds) *Dietary fiber in health and disease*. Plenum Press, New York.

Leeds, A. R. (ed.) (1985) Fibre and diabetes. In: *Fibre perspectives*. John Libbey, London.

Mann, J. I. (1982) *The diabetics diet book: positive health guide.*

Martin Dunitz Ltd, London.

Morgan, L.M., Goulder, T.J., Tsiolakis. D., Marks, V. and Alberti, K.G.M.M. (1979) The effect of unabsorbable carbohydrate on gut hormones. *Diebetologia.* **17**, 85–89.

Paul, A. A. and Southgate, D. A. T. (1978) *McCance and Widdowson's The Composition of Foods*. 4th ed. MRC Special Report Series No.297. HMSO, London.

Rivellese, A., Riccardi, G., Giacco, A., Pacioni, D., Genovese, S., Mattioli, P.L. and Mancini, M. (1980) Effect of dietary fibre on glucose control and serum lipoproteins in diabetic patients. *The Lancet ii*, 447–450.

Simpson, H. C. R., Lousley, S., Geekie, M., Simpson, R. W., Carter, R. D., Hockaday, R. D. R. and Mann, J. I. (1981) A high carbohydrate leguminous fibre diet improves all aspects of diabetic control. *The Lancet i*, 1–5.

Spiller, G. A. and Kay, R. M. (1980) *Medical aspects of dietary fibre*. Plenum Medical Book Co., New York.

Trowell, H., Burkitt, D. and Heaton, K. (1985) *Dietary fibre, fibre-depleted foods and disease*. Academic Press, London.

9

The effects of storage and processing on the nutritional value of food

Ann Walker

Introduction

The purpose of good nutrition is to promote health and general well-being. However, the nutritional quality of food is normally measured in terms of its ability to satisfy human nutrient requirements. Even in the richer nations of the world, the diet may not provide some nutrients at adequate levels for certain groups of people.

The nutrient composition of a food depends on the raw materials, as well as the effects of processing and storage. Some of these effects may be advantageous and render nutrients more biologically available, while others may have a detrimental effect. Potential losses of nutrients as a result of processing and storage are well documented for traditional processes. However, less is known about nutrient loss for newer techniques such as microwave cooking and irradiation, or within the home or institution. Another problem which makes interpretation of the effect of changes on diet difficult is that published data on nutrient loss tend to relate to single food items and rarely to entire diets.

THE NUTRITIONAL ADEQUACY OF THE DIET

The practical significance of the effects of certain food processing techniques on the nutritional value of an individual food must be considered within the context of the diet as a whole. In this section the focus is on the adequacy of the diet — a subject also dealt with in Chapter 1.

To be adequately nourished, in addition to a supply of energy, the human body needs to be supplied with some 40 or so nutrients at specific levels in the diet. Single food items are often judged by their ability to provide all of these nutrients, but in practice they would only be expected to provide part of them in a diet. If the diet provides a nutrient in excess of requirements, then the content of that nutrient in a single food item may be irrelevant. However, if a nutrient is supplied at inadequate or marginal levels in the diet, then care is needed during food processing and storage to ensure its maximum retention.

An assessment of the nutritional adequacy of the diet is normally carried out by comparing the nutrient content of a diet (calculated from data on food intake) with the **Recommended Daily Amount (RDA)** of that nutrient for a specific group of people (DHSS, 1979). While such comparisons cannot be used as evidence that an individual is undernourished (this can only be confirmed with appropriate clinical examination and biochemical testing), it can be used as an indicator that a population may be marginally nourished or undernourished for that nutrient (i.e. it can identify 'at risk' groups).

Data from the National Food Survey (MAFF, 1952 onwards) show that certain nutrients are marginally supplied by the national diet. National Food Survey (NFS) data are derived from averaged intakes for different income groups in different parts of the United Kingdom and are compared with an averaged RDA. For the nation as a whole, values for energy intake are below this RDA, but the NFS does not include food consumed outside the home, so it is likely that energy intake is underestimated. Mean values for iron show that it is only marginally provided in the diet. As these are averaged figures, the implications are that a large number of people may be underprovided with this nutrient in the diet. The situation is worse when households with two or more children are considered: for these, even averaged values for iron from food consumed within the household tend to be below the RDA.

The National Food Survey data are based on records of foods entering households in the UK. To obtain further information on the foods that people eat, it is necessary to examine data obtained from individual weighed dietary surveys. These have been shown to give good reproducibility when carried out with care. Such data, from many parts of the western world, show, for certain human groups, that some nutrients are supplied in the diet in inadequate levels with respect to RDA. Table 9.1 shows the daily intake of some nutrients for 67 British female undergraduates, aged 18–22 years, studying Food Science at Reading University. Data were calculated using *McCance and Widdowson's The Composition of Foods,* (Paul and Southgate, 1978) from a 6-day weighed dietary survey.

Table 9.1 — Daily intake of some nutrients by 67 British female undergraduates aged 18–22 yrs at Reading University from a 6-day weighed dietary survey (1980–1983)

Nutrient	RDA (UK)	Intake of nutrient	
		Mean	Range
Energy (kcal)	2150	1842	927–2710
Calcium (mg)	500	826	333–1310
Iron (mg)	12	11.4	4.7–27.1
Zinc (mg)	15[a]	8.7	3.7–14.9
Thiamin (mg)	0.9	1.1	0.5–2.2
Riboflavin (mg)	1.3	1.7	0.7–5.2
Vitamin C (mg)	30	72	17–208

[a] RDA (USA).

The averaged value for energy intake (Table 9.1) was below the RDA, and the range of values for individuals was wide, extending from 927 to 2710 kcal. This variation in energy intake accounts for some of the variation in the other nutrient intakes, as intake of energy determines intake of other nutrients (Chapter 1). Calcium, thiamin, riboflavin and vitamin C showed averaged intake values above the RDA, but the lowest value of the range was well below the RDA. For iron and zinc even the mean values were below the RDA. As there is no RDA given for zinc in the UK, the value given in Table 9.1 is drawn from the RDA for the USA. Interest in zinc nutrition has increased in recent years, following findings of evidence of zinc deficiency in adolescent males in Iran, and biochemical evidence of zinc deficiency in the USA where the current level of zinc intake is 12.5 mg/head/day.

Nearly three quarters of the foods we eat in the UK are processed in one way or another. As we have seen that some nutrients may not be provided in the diet in adequate amounts for some groups of people, it is important that nutrient retention of food is maximized during processing. For some nutrients, such as protein, which are present in our diets in excess, changes brought about by processing, such as the decreased bioavailability of lysine, are not important from a nutritional point of view. For other nutrients, such as iron and vitamin C, which may be inadequately supplied by diet, it is important to offer food processed in the best possible way to preserve these nutrients.

Nutrient deficiencies caused, for example, by lack of energy or protein in the diet, are usually associated with poorer countries of the Third World and are not normally encountered in industrialized countries. Table 9.2 is a summary of the main nutrients lacking in the diet worldwide. While some of these, such as energy and protein deficiency, are mainly confined to the Third World, others, such as iron deficiency, are worldwide problems.

Vegetarians are an increasingly important group in countries like the UK, but also in many Third World countries for economic reasons. This group (especially vegans – the strict vegetarians) are particularly at risk of lack of vitamins B_{12} and D, which are not found in plant foods and therefore must be supplied in the diet either as supplements (B_{12} for vegans) or made in the body (vitamin D) by the action of sunlight on the skin. Table 9.3 shows good sources of selected nutrients provided by four plant food groups. Although in the western world ovo-lacto vegetarians do not suffer such extreme manifestations of nutrient insufficiency, they can be at risk of iron and calcium deficiency, depending how much they rely on dairy products. A varied, balanced diet should contain adequate amounts of carbohydrate, protein, fat, vitamins and minerals for healthy growth and maintenance. Of these nutrients, vitamins and minerals, which are important for numerous physiological processes in the body, are most susceptible to losses in food preparation. In the Third World, apart from protein-energy malnutrition, all other common primary diseases of malnutrition stem from inadequate vitamin and mineral intakes. For example, the all-too-common deficiency disease, xerophthalmia (causing permanent blindness) is caused by a lack of vitamin A.

EFFECT OF STORAGE ON THE NUTRIENT CONTENT OF FOOD
Storage of plant foods is necessary at harvest, to spread the glut throughout the year. Only foods of low moisture content, like cereals and other grains, or dried fruit, vegetables and tubers can be stored at ambient temperatures. Under poor storage

Table 9.2 — Main nutrients lacking in diets worldwide

Nutrient lack	Group mostly affected	Disease	Countries most affected
Energy/protein	Infants, children	Kwashiorkor, marasmus	T
Iron	Children, women, vegetarians	Anaemia	T/W
Vitamin C[a]	Children, women, elderly	Anaemia	T/W
Iodine	Adults	Goitre	T
	Infants	Cretinism	T
Vitamin D[b]	Children,	Rickets	T
	Vegetarians,	Osteomalacia	T/W
	Elderly women	Osteoporosis [c]	W
Calcium	Pregnant & lactating women	Osteomalacia	T/W
	Elderly	Osteoporosis	W
Vitamin A	Infants	Xerophthalmia (blindness)	T
Folic acid	Children, pregnant women	Anaemia	T/W
Niacin	Maize eaters	Pellagra	T

[a] Vitamin C in the diet aids the absorption of iron. [b] Vitamin D is produced by the skin by the action of sunlight, this is prevented by too much clothing. [c] Osteoporois has a complex aetiology in which low calcium and vitamin D intakes may play a role. T, Third World. W, western world.

Table 9.3 — Good sources of selected nutrients [a] provided by four plant food groups

Food group	Nutrient
Cereals	Energy, protein, dietary fibre [b] vitamin B complex [b], iron [b], calcium [b]
Legumes, oilseeds, nuts	Energy, protein, dietary fibre [b], iron [b], calcium [b], vitamin B complex [b]
Roots	Energy, protein, some vitamin C
Fruit and vegetables	Vitamin C, vitamin A, iron, calcium, vitamin B complex, dietary fibre

[a], nutrients selected may be low in the diets of vulnerable group; [b], particulary high in the hull.

conditions of high temperature and humidity, even with these foods, large losses can occur due to a number of biological agents. In terms of total loss of nutrients, bulk losses in storage can often be more serious than reduction in nutrient content of foods, and, therefore, will be dealt with first.

Bulk losses

Insects, mites and rodents can severely damage food. Losses of seed during storage through insect and rodent infestation may reach as high as 50 % by weight in some countries, particularly in the tropics. Early in storage there may be little evidence of insect infestation, but the population increases logarithmically and in a few months can increase from 1 to 100 000 insects per kg. Typically, the greatest infestation occurs when food supply is short, just before harvest. Although store design, maintenance and hygiene are of the utmost importance, adequate storage facilities will obviously depend on a number of socio-economic factors. The larger producer may be able to afford proper storage facilities, and thus eliminate insect infestation, whereas in rural parts of Africa the subsistence farmer can only minimize insect attack by improvements in traditional storage structures.

As far as rodent control is concerned, methods of control should be aimed at creating storage facilities which do not allow easy access of these animals. Large-scale storage is best in solidly constructed buildings with tight-fitting doors. In the Third World, cribs are usually raised a distance from the ground on supports. By placing cones (usually made from sheet metal) around the supports, with the large side downwards, or by wrapping a thick band of sheet metal around the supports, the crib can be made impenetrable to these animals.

Microorganisms attack grain with a moisture content of about 14 % or above. Moulds (fungi) are capable of producing a wide range of biologically active metabolites, such as those which mimic the female hormone oestrogen. The greatest danger to health is from the mould *Aspergillus flavus*, which, at high ambient temperatures (typical of those found in many tropical countries) can grow on groundnuts and produce the metabolite **aflatoxin**. Although other crops can be affected, it is mainly groundnuts which are of concern in international trade. Aflatoxin has been clearly demonstrated to cause liver cancer in a wide range of experimental and farm animals, and its presence at high levels in the diets of people who live in hot, humid regions of the world has been associated with an extraordinarily high incidence of primary cancer of the liver. (Primary cancer of the liver is normally quite rate in man.) Several well-documented reports show that acute aflatoxin poisoning outbreaks leading to sudden death have occurred in East Africa in recent years and that the problem is increasing. Cooking does not reduce the level of aflatoxin in foods, so it is important that foods be stored with a low enough moisture content to prevent the growth of moulds.

Nutrient losses

One of the great advantages of cereals is that they are easy to store in the seed form and have a low moisture content. Cereals normally dry naturally in the field to a level of moisture which will allow them to be stored for long periods, without spoiling. As long as storage conditions are good and insect infestation is minimized, then there is little loss of nutrients from cereals on storage. However, the whole seeds can be stored for much longer periods of time than the flour, which rapidly deteriorates, especially at high temperatures, as a result of lipid oxidation, which leads to the formation of off-flavours, with loss of antioxidant activity.

Legume storage normally only presents a major problem in the Third World. Legumes are very subject to insect attack by bruchid beetles, and groundnuts in particular are prone to the growth of *A. flavus* (see above), with the development of aflatoxin, so storage conditions are important. Apart from these problems, the longer legume seeds are stored, the longer the time needed to cook them (the **hard-to-cook defect**). As well as the inconvenience this causes, the increased amount of firewood necessary for the long cooking time may impose restrictions on the use of legumes in the Third World where firewood is scarce.

Proper storage conditions will help to delay the occurrence of the hard-to-cook defect. Storage temperatures of less than 10°C are particularly effective, but the costs involved are often prohibitive. Another way to prevent the defect is by adequately drying the seeds before storage. Drying to around 10 % moisture considerably reduces the formation of the hard-to-cook defect on storage, even at high temperatures. However, care should be taken not to over-dry the seeds (<7%), as they will not imbibe water well on soaking (formation of hard shell) and viability of the seed will be diminished. The latter point is particularly important if the seeds are to be used for cultivation.

High moisture foods, such as fruit and leafy vegetables, are perishable and need to be preserved in some way before storage. In many industrialized countries, freezing and canning are commonly used processes, both domestically and commercially. However, in the Third World, the best method of preserving such high moisture foods is **solar drying**: once the moisture content is reduced then the product can be stored at ambient temperatures. Solar drying can be carried out with or without prior blanching (adding to boiling water for 2–4 minutes). Even with blanching, the vitamin C content is lost completely and much of the folic acid, but blanching also destroys spoilage enzymes in the produce, and thus extends the storage life of the product. Vitamin A (carotenes in the case of plant foods) is not greatly affected by blanching or drying, but its activity will decrease in the dried product during prolonged storage.

Some fruits, such as oranges and lemons, may be stored for a considerable time in the fresh state. These fruits are high in vitamin C, but as storage continues, the level will decline gradually, the rate depending on the temperature — the higher the temperature, the more rapidly will the fruit deteriorate. (Successful long-term storage of fruit and vegetables requires a temperature-controlled environment.)

In temperate countries, the main root crop stored is potatoes. The best storage temperature for potatoes is 10°C, as lower temperatures cause starch to be converted to glucose, and higher temperatures lead to rapid sprouting. Potatoes with high sugar content brown easily on cooking owing to Maillard browning and are quite unsuitable for some manufacturing purposes (e.g. chip production).

In tropical countries, roots and tubers generally will not normally store well as they are high in moisture. However, under ambient conditions in the tropics, cassava can be left in the ground to store. This is one of the reasons that cassava has replaced other staples such as yams in many parts of Africa. Unfortunately, this substitution has contributed to protein-energy malnutrition, as cassava is exceptionally low in protein — far lower than the staples it has replaced. To lower the moisture content, root crops like cassava can be sliced or pounded to a flour and sun-dried. Gari, prepared in West Africa from cassava, is one such product. In fact, the production of gari involves a fermentation stage, which results in a slightly acid product, which aids its keeping properties. Some root crops, such as potatoes and yams, contain considerable amounts of vitamin C, but the storage of the roots will lower this content and drying them will remove it all.

A wide range of factors operate during storage and will influence nutrient retention. These include temperature, exposure to light and oxygen, length of time and humidity. While the proximate principles of food (protein, fat, carbohydrate) and minerals are largely unchanged during storage, there will be loss of vitamins at variable rates, depending on the vitamin and the temperature.

Most losses of nutrients are slowed down considerably during **frozen storage** (-18°C), although fat oxidation and some enzymic reaction can still occur slowly. Blanching (short, high-temperature treatment) normally eliminates enzyme reactions during frozen storage. In general, the nutrient content of frozen food is very close to fresh food and can sometimes be higher. For example, peas for freezing are normally harvested and processed very rapidly, whereas peas for sale in greengrocery outlets may be stored at ambient temperatures for several days. Storage, in the retail chain, of fresh vegetables such as peas, can lead to considerable reduction in vitamin C content. For garden peas: 25% loss of vitamin C after one day of storage increasing to 50% loss after four days might be typical figures.

Freezing will normally retain high levels of vitamin C if it is rapidly carried out. Indeed, storage in the frozen condition can retain almost the full value of vitamin C (compared with the recently frozen peas) even for as long as 9 months. Thawing should also be rapid and frozen vegetables are best plunged directly into boiling water.

Canned storage does not greatly affect vitamin C content. Therefore, typically, freshly canned garden peas may contain about 80% of the vitamin C compared with the freshly canned product, from 3 to 9 months after storage, although some of this will be in the brine which will be discarded. Experiments show that there may be an initial drop during early storage and then the level is constant for at least 9 months of storage.

Potatoes are a very important source of vitamin C in Britain, not because the level of vitamin C is exceptionally high, but because potatoes are eaten as such a high proportion of the British diet that they make a significant contribution to the vitamin C content of it. Freshly harvested main crop (old) potatoes might contain about 60 mg/100 g fresh weight. After only 3 months in storage 75% of the vitamin C is lost. Losses after that period of time are much slower. Of course, after that, cooking losses need to be taken into account (see next section).

THE EFFECT OF PROCESSING ON THE NUTRIENT CONTENT OF FOOD

The term **food processing** includes, as well food industry techniques, those techniques applied to food in the home to prepare the food for presentation on the plate. A processed food is thus not easily defined, and might be best considered by those foods excluded, which are fresh fruit and vegetables, eggs, fresh fish and fresh meat. However, even these are normally processed (cooked) in the home before eating. Indeed, many unprocessed foods are unfit for human consumption unless they are processed. For example, cereals are unpalatable and not easily digested, and legumes (peas and beans) contain toxic substances which need to be heat-treated to remove their toxic effects. The following is a summary of the reasons for food processing:

- Storage, preservation
- Prevention of disease
- Improvement of digestibility and nutritive value

- Palatability/acceptability
- Fortification
- Destruction/reduction of toxic components
- To change the physical properties of food.

Food processing enables seasonal foods to be available all year round and allows us access to a wider variety of food. There are many types of processing techniques available, including freezing, drying, heating, evaporating, chilling, fermenting, grinding and mixing. Of all of these, apart from physical methods such as milling and peeling (see below), heat treatment has by far the greatest effect on nutritional value, and therefore most of discussion which follows in this chapter is concerned with this method. Many studies have also focussed on the effects of heating on vitamin retention. This is because some vitamins, in particular vitamin C and perhaps thiamin, readily undergo chemical reactions which reduce the vitamin activity. For this reason vitamin losses after heat treatment are used as an indicator of processing change, on the assumption that if vitamin losses are acceptable, then other nutrients will be largely retained.

The effects of processing are normally considered in terms of their detrimental effects on the nutrient composition of food. There are, however, some beneficial effects. Foods are processed to improve their sensory qualities, to destroy pathogenic organisms and for preservation purposes. At the same time, the nutritional quality may be increased by improved digestibility of (a) starch, owing to gelatinization and of (b) protein, owing to denaturation and destruction of toxic substances. Heat degradation of the cell walls of plant foods may lead to increased availability of nutrients such as carotenoids (pro-vitamin A).

Other forms of processing which have beneficial effects on nutritional quality of foods are **fermentation,** which is known to increase the content of B complex vitamins, and **seed germination,** which leads to increased vitamin C content of grains, including legumes. Dry seeds contain no vitamin C, but 3 days after germination, legume seeds contain as much as cabbage, which is considered to be a good source (see Fig. 9.1). It is said that, long before the discovery that scurvy could be cured on the long European sea voyages (see Chapter 3) by adding fruit to the diet, the Chinese sailors used to take seeds for sprouting in pots to avoid this condition on long voyages!

The detrimental effects of processing on the nutritional quality of food are:

Loss of major components

- Bulk (weight) (by milling, peeling, leaching)
- Dietary fibre (by milling, peeling)
- Protein quality (excessive heat treatment only)
- Sugars (leaching)
- Acceptability (through rancidity caused by lipid oxidation)

Loss of Minor Components

- Water-soluble vitamins (by milling, peeling, leaching, oxidation, heat instability)
- Fat-soluble vitamins (by heat instability, oxidation)
- Minerals (by milling, peeling)

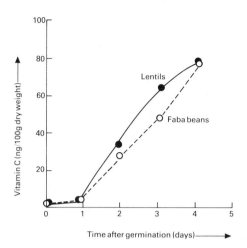

Fig. 9.1 — Effect of germination on vitamin C content of two legumes. Data from Hsu *et al.*, 1980.

The most important losses on processing are of:

- Bulk (weight) (through milling, peeling)
- Dietary fibre
- Water-soluble vitamins.

Bulk (weight) loss may be considerable for some processes but often these losses are inadequately reported in the literature. Bulk loss is of considerable importance with respect to cereals, which still provide a large proportion of the diet in the industrialized world — about one third of the total energy of the diet in the UK. Therefore, because of the large quantities eaten, loss of nutrients as a result of **milling** of cereals has a large effect on the overall nutrient content of the diet. Besides loss of niacin, thiamin, iron and calcium, which are made up by nutrient restoration in most countries, there is a large loss of dietary fibre. Fig. 9.2 shows the nutrient and fibre losses of wheat flour of different extraction rates (100% extraction is wholemeal, while 72% is 'white' flour). The importance to health, in particular to gut function, of retaining dietary fibre in cereal foods has become apparent over recent years.

After the removal of the hull, milling is continued for most cereals in order to produce flour. This process will induce more rapid oxidation of lipids and antioxidants, but starch in flour will be gelatinised more readily during cooking or baking than starch in the whole seed, and this will make it more digestible, as starches from some cereals (and tubers) are not very digestible in the raw, uncooked state.

Legumes are **dehulled** in many parts of the Third World by milling or pounding in a pestle and mortar (after the addition of a little water). This is a common treatment prior to cooking. For coloured beans, dehulling reduces the content of tannins, as these are

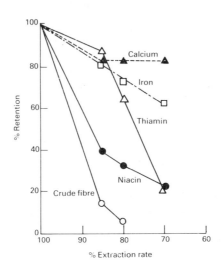

Fig. 9.2 — Relationship between extraction rate and retention of some nutrients in wheat flour.

confined to the seed coat, and this will improve digestibility. It is unlikely that dehulling will have any marked effect on the level of other toxic materials, as they are mostly found in the cotyledons of the seed. The main effect of dehulling on the nutritional value is to reduce the amount of calcium, which is concentrated in the hull. This source of calcium is very important for vegans and many Third World populations.

In the Third World, loss of thiamin (B_1) can be very significant in the preparation of polished (milled) rice (Table 9.4). In the past the low level of thiamin in polished rice has led to many cases of beri-beri (Chapters 3 and 5). More recently, cases of beri-beri have reappeared among Japanese teenagers with unbalanced diets high in white rice and soft drinks. The higher the carbohydrate contribution to the diet, the greater the requirement for thiamin. Parboiling (a steaming treatment before milling) does improve the thiamin content of polished rice to some extent.

For roots and tubers, preparation for eating (other than cooking), normally involves the removal of the peel, which is high in dietary fibre and vitamin C. To retain as much of the vitamin as possible, either the roots should be cooked and eaten with the scrubbed peel left on, or the peel should be removed as thinly as possible.

The **outer leaves** of leafy vegetables are often discarded although they have the highest vitamin C and carotene contents. As a general rule, dark green leaves contain more carotene (pro-vitamin A) and vitamin C than paler ones. Indeed, carotenoids are accessory pigments to chlorophyll and help it to harness energy from sunlight. In general, the greater the amounts of chlorophyll in a leaf, the greater the amounts of carotenoids. **Cutting** fruit and vegetables releases an enzyme, ascorbase, which acts rapidly on vitamin C to break it down and render it useless as a nutrient. Figure 9.3 shows the

Table 9.4 — Composition of rice before and after milling

	Carbohydrate %	Protein %	Fat %	Mineral content %	Vit. B$_1$ mg/100 g
Brown Rice	86	8.7–9.9	2.3	1.2–2.1	0.4
Milled Rice	90	6.7–8.6	0.3	0.4–0.9	0.1 [a]

[a], rice milled after parboiling has a vitamin B$_1$ content of 0.15 – 0.2 mg/100 g

breakdown and excretion products of vitamin C in the body and its degradation in foods. Therefore, cutting fruit and vegetables should be done as close as possible to the time of eating or cooking. Vegetables prepared for salads or for cooking should not be cut too fine, as the greater the amount of cutting, the greater the release of ascorbase. In addition, the greater the amount of cutting, the greater the surface area from which vitamin C (and other water-soluble vitamins and minerals) can be lost into washing or cooking water (leaching). To minimise loss, fruit and vegetables should be washed before cutting, not after.

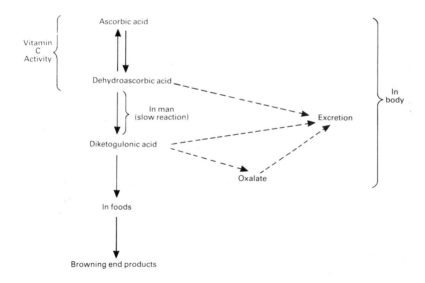

Figure 9.3 — Metabolism of Vitamin C in the body and its degradation in foods.

From ancient times, **alkaline salts** have been added to the cooking water of leafy vegetables (to improve the colour) and to legumes to shorten the cooking time. These salts may be naturally occurring, or purchased as sodium bicarbonate. In any case, the practice of adding alkaline salts is to be discouraged as it will inactivate vitamin C (high in vegetables) and thiamin (high in legumes). The loss of thiamin is of particular concern when legumes accompany white rice, which is also very low in thiamin. To reduce the long cooking time of legumes, pressure cooking should be encouraged as this reduces the demand on scarce fuel resources.

Heat treatment is particularly important in the preparation of legumes for consumption, as it not only destroys many toxic substances, but also ensures the preparation of a palatable food. The toxic substances, haemagglutinins (lectins) and trypsin inhibitors are proteins and can be inactivated by heat. However, the time needed to remove their effects depends on a number of factors, such as moisture, temperature and particle size. Other toxic substances are not removed by cooking. These include favism factors responsible for causing favism if broad beans (*Vicia faba*) are eaten by susceptible people.

Fruit and vegetables should be cooked in the minimum amount of water for the shortest possible time to prevent **leaching** and thus retain water-soluble vitamins. Cooking at boiling temperatures destroys ascorbase and prevents the rapid breakdown of vitamin C. Thus, chopped vegetables retain more vitamin C if they are placed directly into a minimum quantity of boiling water, rather than into cold water which is then brought to the boil. Therefore, rather than completely submerging vegetables in water for cooking, put only 1–2 cm of water into a saucepan and bring to the boil before adding the vegetables, then cook with the lid on. This method effectively cooks the food by steaming. The cooking liquid will contain valuable water-soluble nutrients which can be made into sauces.

During heating, the amino acid lysine can react with reducing sugars such as glucose in the non-enzymic browning reaction (the **'Maillard' reaction**). This type of reaction is responsible for the brown colour of toast for example. In mild heating, losses of lysine are negligible, but they can be marked if heating is severe. However, this loss is very unlikely to be of great nutritional significance to most people eating a varied diet, as intakes of protein, even in poor situations, are normally quite adequate and well above requirements.

As most drying operations are perfomed in the presence of oxygen, vitamin destruction, particularly of **vitamin C** would be expected. Instant mashed potatoes are manufactured by drying techniques and the loss of vitamin C in the process is made good by subsequent addition of vitamin C to the final product. Some vitamin C of fruit and vegetable is retained on canning, but the amount is variable and depends on the canning conditions. Certainly, no one should rely on the vitamin C content of canned fruit or vegetables to provide their main source of this nutrient.

It might be thought that there would be masses of good data on the effects of processing on the nutritional value of food. Although the literature is scattered with experiments on individual food items, not all this information is directly relevant to the 'on the plate' situation. Unfortunately, a lot of comparisons of raw material versus processed material do not compare like with like. Sometimes, long periods of storage of the processed product may not be taken into account. Fresh vegetables may be compared directly with frozen vegetables, although the starting material may be quite different and no account is taken of the fact that to present the food 'on the plate' the fresh vegetable might have to be cooked twice as long as the blanched, frozen product.

Predicting nutrient loss in food processing

In recent years, attempts have been made to formulate mathematical relationships to enable prediction and optimization of nutrient retention during thermal processing. So far these mathematical relationships have found little practical use owing to a number of factors. Table 9.5 summarizes the various problems of predicting nutrient loss due to processing.

Table 9.5— Problems of predicting nutrient loss due to processing

- The nutrient content of raw materials is variable

- Existing assay method may be unsuitable or cumbersome for quality control purposes

- The nutrient may not be present in a single form → analytical problems

- Nutrients may be degraded by a number of mechanisms, each proceeding at a different rate and influenced differently by reaction conditions

- For nutrients which are degraded by enzymes, enzyme inactivation must also be considered

- Some nutrients may be protected from degradation within specific food products by other components

- It is difficult to measure exact temperature/time relationships for the process

Firstly, there is the wide **variability in composition** of raw materials. For example, the vitamin C contents of canned tomato juice can vary from about 2 to 20 mg/100 g, depending on batch and year of harvest. While some of this variability, particularly for the vitamin C, may be accounted for by differences in the processing conditions, a large part is due to variability of the composition of raw tomato juice. This is emphasized by the wide range of values for carotene found in canned tomato juice (the levels of carotene are not greatly affected by thermal processing).

Secondly, analytical problems may also make prediction of nutrient loss due to processing difficult. While established **analytical methods** for some vitamins may be relatively straightforward, others, such as that for folic acid or vitamin D, were cumbersone in the past. Although vitamin analysis has undergone something of a comeback in recent years, particularly with the introduction of high-pressure liquid chromatography (HPLC) techniques, much research is still needed to make these methods robust and reproducible before they are suitable to be used as routine quality control measures in industry, by relatively unskilled technicians. To complicate matters for the analyst, **a number of different chemical forms of a nutrient** may be present in foods (Table 9.6), each having a different nutrient potency.

Table 9.6 — Substances contributing to nutrient activity

Nutrient	Substance
Vitamin C	Ascorbic acid dehydroascorbic acid
Vitamin B_6	Pyridoxine pyridoxal pyridoxamine
Niacin	Nicotinic acid tryptophan
Vitamin E	8 tocopherols tocotrienols
Vitamin A	Retinol retinal retinoic acid β-carotene γ-carotene α-carotene
Methionine	Methionine cystine (partly)
Phenylalanine	Phenylalanine tyrosine (partly)

Thirdly, **nutrients may be degraded by more than one mechanism**, each proceeding at a different rate and influenced differently by reaction conditions. If the nutrient is degraded by an enzyme, as ascorbic acid is by ascorbase, then enzyme inactivation must also be considered. Some **nutrients may be protected from degradation** within specific food products by other components. Thus, folates are often found in combined forms which are biologically active and more stable than the free form.

Although prediction of nutrient loss is not an easy matter, empirical studies have shown that because of the close relationship between the temperature dependence of quality factors such as colour, texture, vitamins and flavour, processes optimized for sensory quality attributes (taste, smell, texture, etc.) are also optimal for nutrient retention. In most industrialized countries, food processing practice is already optimized for sensory characteristics; therefore, one would not expect to be able to bring about large improvements in nutritional quality by changing processing conditions. However, slight improvements can result from modifications based on optimization techniques, as shown with studies to compare nutrient retention in retort pouch techniques with conventional canning (see below). Generally, in thermal processing, the use of higher temperature, shorter time processes results in greater nutrient retention.

To **estimate nutritional losses** the best approach is to consider the general points affecting loss of a particular nutrient. For example, vitamins are affected differently by prevailing conditions, and Table 9.7 summarizes some of the various factors which affect the stability of vitamins in food. Leaching is a process which leads to considerable loss of minerals and water-soluble vitamins. As far as heat processing is concerned, the most important chemical changes from a nutritional point of view are those occurring in vitamins. Some vitamins are more heat-labile than others; in particular thiamin is very susceptible in this respect. Loss of vitamin activity may also depend on the amount of oxygen present in the foodstuff (for vitamin A and C) or the amount of exposure to light (for riboflavin and to some extent vitamins A and C). The vitamin C content of fruit and vegetables is often used to monitor the effects of various processes. The combined effects of enzyme degradation and susceptibility to oxidation and leaching make the vitamin C content of foods particularly vulnerable to processing.

Table 9.7 — Some factors affecting the stability of certain vitamins in food

Vitamin	Solubility	Subject to oxidation	Heat-labile	Light-sensitive
Vitamin A	No	Yes	No	Slight
Riboflavin	Yes	No	No	Yes
Thiamin	Yes	No	Yes	No
Vitamin C	Yes	Yes	No	Slight

Therefore, nutrient loss will very much depend on raw materials used in manufacturing, and conditions prevailing at the time of manufacture, including time and temperature, recipe, amount of stirring etc. Precise information on nutrient losses in food manufacture can only by obtained be extensive studies (over a number of batches) of the actual product. However, manufacturers (and indeed consumers) can obtain guidelines on nutrient loss by studying data obtained under experimental conditions. Throughout the literature there are many examples showing the effects of processing, especially thermal processing, on the retention of vitamins in foods. Table 9.8 gives one such example, in which a comparison is made between frozen/cooked and canned vegetables for water-soluble vitamins. The canning process leads to greater mean loss of vitamins than freezing followed by cooking, but for each mean value there is a wide range of values.

Another approach used to estimate vitamin loss is to use the approximate corrections used in *McCance and Widdowson's The Composition of Foods* (Paul and Southgate, 1978). These values are given in Figure 9.4, but it must be remembered, in the light of the previous discussion, that these are very approximate figures and losses can vary considerably if conditions are much different from those under which this data was collected.

As well as the points mentioned in Table 9.5 which make nutrient loss on processing difficult to predict, the method of heating will also affect nutrient loss depending on:
● stability of nutrient
● size and type of food

• container used
• heating rate of equipment
• handling required during heating, e.g. stirring, exposure to air or light.

Table 9.8 — Losses of vitamins from vegetables during canning and freezing

Processing	No. of vegetables examined		Loss of vitamins compared to fresh-cooked (%)			
			Thiamin	Riboflavin	Niacin	Vit. C
Frozen boiled, drained	10	Mean	20	24	24	26
		Range	0–61	0–45	0–56	0–78
Canned drained	7	Mean	67	42	49	51
		Range	56–83	14–50	31–65	28–67

Source: *Food Technology* (1977) **31** (12), 32–38

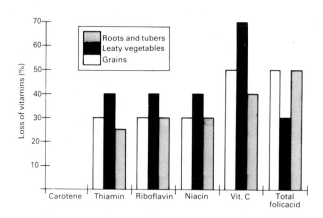

Fig. 9.4 — Percentage losses of vitamins from plant foods during cooking. Data from Paul and Southgate, 1978.

As an example of this, Fig. 9.5 shows the vitamin retention of sweet potato puree processed in a retort pouch compared with a conventional can. There is very little difference in the levels of β-carotene of these two treatments, as this is a relatively heat-stable substance, but there are increased retentions of both thiamin and riboflavin using the retort pouch, which required a shorter retorting time in order to achieve commercial sterility.

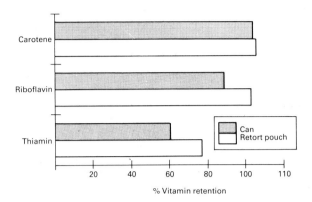

Fig. 9.5 — Vitamin retention in sweet potato puree processes in two types of container to $F_0 = 8.0 \pm$ 0.3 min at 121.1°C. Data from Rizvi and Acton, 1982. F_0 refers to equivalent heating time at 121.1°C.

Nutrient loss in recently developed processing methods

In recent years many of the traditional processes have been modified to increase (for example, speed of production, or to give better hygiene standards. These new methods include shorter-time canning techniques (see Fig. 9.5), aseptic processing, irradiation, slow cookers, 'boil-in-bag' techniques and various continuous steamers, fryers and cookers for large-scale catering. Two very interesting and novel approaches to food preservation and processing involve the use of electromagnetic radiation: irradiation, using γ-rays, X- rays or electron beams and microwave processing and cooking. While a considerable amount of data exists on the processing losses of nutrients due to well-established commercial practices such as canning and freezing, less information is available on the vitamin losses due to recently developed techniques. The studies which do exist usually compare the new technique with a more conventional method.

As far as *microwave cooking* is concerned, the main advantage of this process is that vegetables (and other foods) can be cooked with very little or no water. This cuts down the time of cooking and also reduces leaching losses of minerals and water-soluble vitamins. The importance of leaching is well illustrated in Table 9.9, which gives data on a comparison of microwave cooking with conventional cooking of peas. There was no advantage with respect to total ascorbic acid retention if the same amount of water was used for both forms of cooking. However, microwave cooking did show an advantage if the peas were cooked without added water.

The advantages of microwave cooking in the retention of vitamin C perhaps best illustrate the use of this technique in vitamin conservation. But there are also some small advantages for other vitamins as well. Although experiments show that very little folate is lost from, for example spinach cooked either conventionally or in a microwave oven, there is an advantage of microwave cooking over roasting in a conventional oven at 204°C for thiamin retention for broiler chicken.

On the whole, it is not easy from the literature to come to a consistent view of the effects of microwaving on the nutrient retention of foods. Comparisons of this method of cooking with other methods are not well controlled in many of the experiments, and before 1960, when many of these studies were carried out, the oven specifications were

Table 9.9 — Vitamin C content of peas (400 g) cooked by different methods

Treatments[a]	Total ascorbic acid (%) retention on dry basis)
None	100
Conventional cooking (simmered with 100g water, 8.0 min)	77.7
Microwave[b] cooking (100g water, 8.0 min)	76.7
Microwave cooking (no water, 6.5 min)	87.2

[a] vessels covered; [b] 115V domestic.
Adapted from: Mabesa and Baldwin, 1979.

not mentioned. However, the general consensus of opinion seems to be that microwave cooked food is, in general, likely to be comparable in nutrient composition to the equivalent food cooked conventionally. More recently, there has been concern that some microwave cookers do not heat foods evenly and that considerable temperature gradients can exist. This is the subject of on-going study by MAFF (Ministry of Agriculture, Fisheries and Food, UK). Recent reports that microwaving of foods containing proteins cause detrimental amino acid isomerism appear to be ill-founded.

Food irradiation is a controversial technique, which has now been cleared for use on a limited basis in many western countries. The technique has been the subject of very extensive toxicological testing, which has shown safety for consumption of foods that have received dose levels up to 1 Mrad (10 kGy). However, the consumer perception of irradiation is linked with the suspicion of presence of radioactive residues in the food, which would be potentially harmful to health. However, there is no evidence of increased radioactivity levels in foods after irradiation (DHSS, 1986).

Despite consumer resistance, it is likely that in future at least limited use of irradiation may extend to pathogen decontamination of food ingredients, such as spices, and insect disinfestation of grains. The reason is that high pathogen counts of spices are a potential source of a much greater hazard — e.g. Salmonella which may lead to high counts in food manufacturing. Irradiation applied to spices may also result in a reduction in levels of bacterial spores such as *Clostridium botulinum*, although permitted dose levels may not eliminate all spores. The alternative method of insect disinfestation, which is used at the moment, is to use fumigants, which leave behind residues in the food chain.

Other uses of irradiation such as the prolongation of storage life of certain fruit, meat and fish under refrigerated conditions, inhibition of sprouting of potatoes or growth of mushrooms and inactivation of *Salmonella* in meat, poulty and egg products are likely to be more contentious issues, and consumer opinion may well preclude its use. However, some consumers may welcome the choice of reducing pathogen hazard by eating irradiated foods, particularly prawns and poultry products. Questions of proper labelling

of irradiated products, licencing of premises for food irradiation and Good
Manufacturing Practice (GMP) for the technique are still under discussion.

High levels of radiation cause chemical changes in food, and it is the production of
these free radicals, which are short-lived but highly-reactive chemicals, that is of
particular concern (antioxidants and free radicals are dealt with briefly in Chapter 7).
Complete sterilization of foods, including destruction of bacterial spores, requires doses
up to 5 Mrad and at these levels there is distinct off-flavour production and considerable
nutrient destruction. However, at the levels specified for use with foods, nutrient losses
due to irradiation up to 1 Mrad (10 kGy) are mostly small, although some concern has
been expressed at the high losses of vitamin C in stored, irradiated potatoes. Fig. 9.6
shows the effect of irradiation of 0.6 Mrad on three vitamins in cod. Thiamin is
particularly susceptible to degradation by irradiation, as can be seen from Figure 9.6.

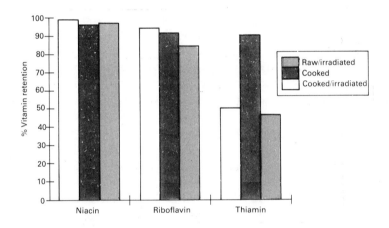

Figure 9.6 — Effect of γ-radiation (0.6 Mrad) and cooking (4 min) on three B-complex vitamins
in cod. Data from *Journal of the Science of Food and Agriculture* (1971) **22**, 146–148.

Data are also presented in Fig. 9.6 on the combined effect on cod of γ-radiation,
followed by cooking. The cooking step has a greater effect on the riboflavin content of
cod than γ-radiation, while the reverse is true for thiamin for this food.

NUTRIENT LOSS IN THE FOOD CHAIN

It is rare to find data (as given in Fig. 9.6) in the literature dealing with the effects of
more than one process, despite the fact that, either in the food factory or in the home,
food eaten may have been subjected to a number of processes such as canning and
reheating or freezing and stewing.

On the whole, food eaten in the home contains nutrients at predictable levels, as
found in a recent survey of 23 healthy elderly people living in their own homes. This

study showed that for a large number of foods, including cooked samples, analysed values for vitamin C contents of foods were close to values taken from food tables. The same is not true for institutional catering, as the vitamin C contents of foods taken from the British food tables overestimate the vitamin C content of foods prepared in this way.

An increasing proportion of meals are eaten outside the home in the western world. In 1980 in the UK, 13% of the money spent on food was spent outside the home. The combined effect of various processes on nutrient retention is particularly important in institutional catering, where so many steps are involved. Large losses of vitamins can occur in catering, especially if there is a tendency to overcook or to hold food at high temperatures for long times. If vegetables are kept hot for several hours, then they will be almost devoid of vitamin C as well as sustaining losses of other vitamins. At the same time, there is also loss of sensory quality. While conventional cooking of food from fresh is still used for catering purposes, with food held warm after cooking, until served, cook/chill/reheat and cook/freeze/reheat operations have been introduced and these, if done properly, improve nutrient retention.

A group of American researchers identified the steps in food preparation which caused largest nutrient loss in a simulated hospital cook/chill catering system. They monitored the thiamin retention in beef loaf and peas and the ascorbic acid content of potatoes. Largest nutrient losses were found for beef loaf in the precooking step, for peas at reheating and for potatoes in the 24h chilled storage.

Even greater losses of nutrients may occur during the delivery of hot meals, especially if considerable delay occurs between preparation and serving. This is exemplified by data from three services providing 'meals on wheels' in Leeds (UK) which were analysed for their vitamin C content. Reductions in vitamin C content of around 50% (compared with the freshly prepared food) were recorded on average for the last meal served.

'HEALTHY' EATING AND NEW FOOD PRODUCTS

With the publication of the COMA (1984) Report (Chapter 1) and its recommendations for dietary change, there has been a flurry of activity among food manufacturers to produce alternative products to meet consumer demand for low saturated fat, low sugar, low salt products. The use of nutrition by the food industry in product development and marketing is described in full in Chapter 10. Some examples are given here of the way in which the food industry can effect very great changes in food composition.

Although the lowering of salt content of food may only be an advantage to a certain proportion of the population, in respect of high blood pressure, nevertheless, food manufacturers have been looking at ways of reducing salt in manufactured food. Table 9.10 shows the sodium content of some traditionally processed foods, with their raw materials, showing the very large quantities of sodium which have be added in the past. Recently, attempts have been made to reduce the sodium content of manufactured foods; the salt content of bread is being gradually reduced so that people will get used to the taste of low-salt bread. Many canned vegetables are now being produced without any added sodium, so the levels should now be comparable with the raw materials. Table 9.10 also shows how great the scope is for reducing the sodium content of some breakfast cereals, which have as much as 1.7 g/100 g of sodium, compared to others which only have 4.0 mg/100 g!

Table 9.10 — Sodium content of some raw and processed foods

Food	Method of processing	Sodium content (mg/100 g)
Flour	All extractions	2.0–4.0
	Self raising	350
Bread	All types	540–580
Breakfast cereals		4.0–1670
Butter	Unsalted	7.0
	Salted	870
Beef	Raw	49
	Corned	870
Peas	Fresh, raw	1
	Canned	230

Source: Paul and Southgate, 1978.

Food manufacturing has greatly influenced the range of yellow fats on the market over recent years. Apart from low-fat spreads, which can be used in energy-reduced diets (Chapter 6), margarines with good spreading ability straight from the refrigerator have been developed (soft margarines). These have the nutritional advantage that they are also high in PUFA (polyunsaturated fatty acids), the intake of which has been recommended by COMA (1984) to replace a reduction of hard fats, like butter. Fig. 9.7 shows the saturated, monounsaturated and polyunsaturated proportions of butter, hard margarine and a typical soft margarine.

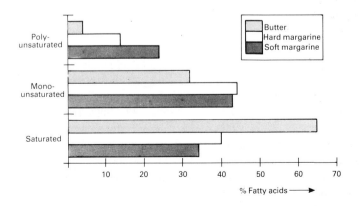

Fig. 9.7 — Saturated and unsaturated fatty acids in butter and margarine. From Paul, 1977.

The food industry for many years has been responsible for adding nutrients to foods in food manufacture, which will change their nutritional value. Sometimes these additions are made in order to make a claim about the nutritional value, as in the case of vitamins and minerals added to breakfast cereals. At other times nutrients may be added for some technical reason, for example, vitamin C can be used as an antioxidant to prevent early browning of fruit juices and thus extend shelf life. Table 9.11 shows some examples of nutrient addition to foods in the UK. Calcium has been added to white flour since the last World War, in order to bring it up to the nutritional value of wholemeal flour. Despite the fact that the national diet is now high in dairy products and on the whole adequately supplied with calcium, this practice is continued, particularly as there is some indication that high levels of calcium may protect against coronary heart disease (the incidence of coronary heart disease in hard water areas is lower than in soft water areas — see Chapter 7).

Table 9.11 —Examples of nutrient addition to foods

Nutrient	Food	Reasons for addition
Vitamins A & D	Margarine	Compulsory enrichment
Calcium	White flour	Compulsory restoration/ enrichment
Iron, thiamin & niacin	White flour Breakfast cereals	Compulsory restoration Voluntary enrichment
Dietary fibre	Breakfast cereals	Voluntary enrichment
Vitamin C	Fruit juices, squashes	Antioxidant
β-carotene	Margarine, jellies, etc	Colouring agent
Vitamin E	Cooking oils	Antioxidant

CONCLUSION

A number of surveys have shown that, even in our highly technological society, a large proportion of the population may be below the RDA for some nutrients. In institutional catering this may be further exacerbated for nutrients such as vitamin C which are susceptible to oxidation during long, heated holding periods. Patients in hospitals often have increased requirements for certain nutrients after surgery to ensure a speedy recovery and these may not be met in the food provided. Food provided by the food industry in the western world has never been more varied, but there is no room for complacency and we must continue to strive to provide food of as high a standard of nutritional quality as possible. Improvements in storage facilities and in food cooking and preparation techniques and the introduction of appropriate technologies to facilitate cooking and shorten cooking time, would lead to better nutritional value of food.

REFERENCES

Bender, A. E. (1978) *Food processing and nutrition*. Academic Press, London.

DHSS (Department of Health and Social Security) (1979) *Recommended Daily Amounts of food energy and nutrients for groups of people in the United Kingdom*. Report on Health and Social Subjects No. 15. HMSO, London.

DHSS (1984) *Diet and cardiovascular disease*. The 'COMA Report'. Report on Health and Social Subject No. 28. HMSO, London.

DHSS (1986) *Report on the safety and wholesomeness of irradiated foods*. Advisory Committee on irradiated and novel foods. HMSO, London.

Harris, R. S. and Karmas, E. (eds) (1975) (1975) *Nutritional evaluation of food processing*. Avi Publishing Co Inc, Westport Connecticut, USA.

Hsu, D., Leung, H.K., Finney, P.L. and Morad, M.M. (1980) Effect of germination on nutritive value and baking properties of dry peas, lentils and faba beans. *Journal of Food Science*, **45**, 87–92

Mabesa, L.B. and Baldwin, R.E. (1979) Ascorbic acid in peas cooked by microwaves. *Journal of Food Science*, **44**, 932

MAFF (Ministry of Agriculture, Fisheries and Food) (1952 onwards) *Household food consumption and expenditure*. Annual Reports of the National Food Survey Committee. HMSO, London.

Paul, A.A. (1977) Changes in food composition. *British Nutrition Foundation Nutrition Bulletin*, **4**(3). 173.

Paul, A. A. and Southgate, D. A. T. (1978) *McCance and Widdowson's The Composition of Foods*. 4th ed. MRC Special Report No. 297. HMSO, London.

Rechcigl Jnr, M. (1982) *Handbook of nutritive value of processed food*. Vol. 1. CRC Press Inc, Florida, USA.

Rizvi, S.S.H. and Action, J.C. (1982) Nutrient enhancement of thermostabilized food in retort pouches. *Food Technology*, **36**(4). 105.

Walker, A. F. (1984) The nutritional quality of food. In: Birch, G. G. and Parker, K. J. (eds) Control of food quality and food analysis. Elsevier Applied Science Publishers, London.

10

Nutrition and the food industry
David Richardson

Introduction
Major changes in the food market and in patterns of food consumption indicate that people are increasingly interested in health, diet and nutrition. Consumers are prepared to change long-established eating habits if particular foods or ingredients are perceived to be 'unhealthy' and acceptable alternatives are available.

The increased awareness of nutrition has led to more consumer demand for more information about the foods they eat. Concern over diet and health, changing eating habits and family meal patterns, newer and quicker methods of preparing foods, together with increasing retailer and government interest in the 'wholesomeness' of foods have become real issues which are influencing the purchase decision. These factors, in turn, are affecting sales of existing food items and new product developments.

Extensive research and technological developments in the food industry have made possible a vast range of products which fill our shops and supermarkets. Fewer than half of these products existed in the UK 10–20 years ago. Examples include products such as frozen cakes and pastries, canned maize, pizzas, coffee creamers, fruit-flavoured yoghurts, lasagne, soya dishes and extruded savoury snacks. Whether the new products are successful or not depends very much on the quality of the product, and this term is defined rather differently by the producer and by the consumer, as shown in Table 10.1.

For the consumer, the demand for various foods is inextricably bound up with their availability, price, convenience, and attraction, in terms of colour, taste, and 'food appeal'. The last term is perhaps best described as the individual's psychological and social assessment of the appropriateness of the product in the context of his/her lifestyle (Plate 10.1). For the manufacturer, a key issue is to ensure as far as possible that the product is going to be profitable and generate cash rather than consume it. The quality definitions for the producer, therefore, are associated more closely with the composition, flavour and texture of the product, its stability, its safety and packaging in relation to costs. The overall objective of the food manufacturer are to provide the consumer with a wide choice of quality foods and to pay particular attention to the factors which are embodied in the IFST Guidelines *Food and the Public Interest*, the outlines of which are given in Table 10.2.

Table 10.1 — Quality definitions as seen by producers and consumers of food

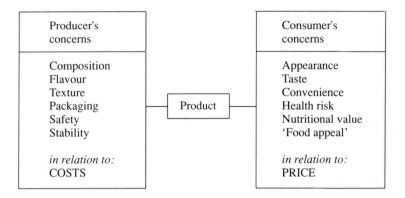

Producer's concerns		Consumer's concerns
Composition		Appearance
Flavour		Taste
Texture		Convenience
Packaging	Product	Health risk
Safety		Nutritional value
Stability		'Food appeal'
in relation to:		*in relation to:*
COSTS		PRICE

Table 10.2 — Summary of IFST guidelines on food and the public interest

Supply:	that there is and continues to be a sufficient amount of food, with healthy and efficient production and distributive industries capable of supplying it.
Variety:	that there is sufficient variety to enable people to choose the kinds, forms and versions of food they prefer, etc.
Wholesomeness:	that the food is wholesome and its manufacture and handling is carried out to ensure maximum quality, stability and safety.
Nourishment:	that although most people tend to choose a wide variety of foods nevertheless diets based substantially on manufactured foods can provide enough of the right kinds of nourishment for energy and good health.
Economy:	that manufactured foods are prepared and distributed as efficiently and economically as possible.
Information:	that the public is adequately enabled to know what it is buying and what measures/precaution should be taken in storing and using it.
Redress:	that adequate resource exists for a purchaser to seek and obtain appropriate redress in the case of justifiable complaint.

IFST, Institute of Food Science and Technology (UK)
Adapted from Blanchfield, 1980.

NUTRITION AND FOOD PRODUCT DEVELOPMENT

In the past, the criteria for screening a new product idea have tended to be marketing factors, and questions asked have included:

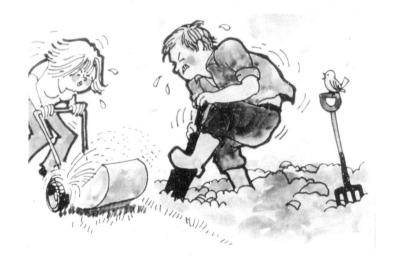

Plate 10.1 — 'Food appeal' is concerned with an individual's psychological and social assessment of the appropriateness of a food product in the context of his or her lifestyle.

Does the product idea fit into the company's strategy?
Does the product idea satisfy a consumer need?
Is the market segment big enough to build a business on?
Do we have the resources to counter a competitive response?
What are the costs of development and introduction?

All these fundamental commercial questions allow management to assess the scale of risk and investment involved in the introduction of a new product, the need for test markets and the decision to launch. The marketing strategy usually involves an advertising campaign, which includes items such as the finalization of the product name; agreement on what advertising claims are to be used; the completion of advertising copy for television, radio, newspapers, magazines and coupons, etc; the determination of label artwork and the final package design; and assessment of the product quality attributes which are to be conveyed to the consumer.

Working in close collaboration with marketing, the responsibilities of the technical team for ensuring the safety, quality and nutritional value of food products are shown in Table 10.3. In brief, the manufacturer must not only know the technology of combining ingredients to produce an attractive, palatable and safe food, but in the current regulatory climate, give serious consideration to the formulation, labelling and cost implications of the existing and proposed food regulations. Table 10.4 outlines the basis of quality assurance in the food industry.

Table 10.3 — The technical team's responsibility for ensuring the safety, quality and nutritional value of foods.

- Product formulation

- Processing parameters

- Claims documentation

- Ingredient declaration
  /nutrition labelling

- Storage stability development –
  e.g. N_2 flushing

- Packaging

- Specifications – raw materials,
  semi-finished and finished products

- Recipe — the preperation and cooking
  instructions — especially for
  microwave products

Table 10.4 — Quality assurance procedures used by the food industry to demonstrate 'due diligence' and care to supply safe, quality foods

The Procedures are based on:

- Purchasing specifications

- Manufacturing standards

- Programme of sampling and analysis
  of raw materials and finished products

- Ensuring freedom from contamination
  during manufacture, storage and
  distribution

Manufacturers, therefore, require expert advice very early on in new product development and throughout all the stages to launch (Plate 10.2). Expertise in food labelling has become as important an issue to product development as any marketing or processing factor, and early advice can avoid costly mistakes and make sure that the

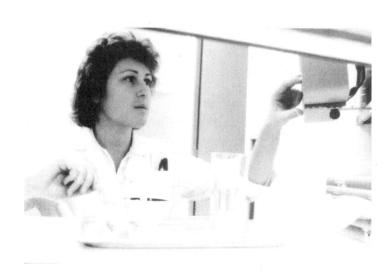

Plate. 10.2 — Manufacturers require expert advice (seen here in sensory evaluation) very early on in
new food product development and throughout all stages to launch.

company, or the individual managers, are not violating the law. Basically, the law
requires that any food product must conform to its description; it must also be of
merchantable quality, and be fit for use. The prime consideration of all the rules and
codes of practice on labelling is to inform and protect the consumer, and increasingly to
fulfil an educational and a reassuring role.

As the introduction of any new product requires assessment and consideration of a
whole range of regulatory, marketing and technical points, further questions need to be
researched such as:

— Do the ingredient suppliers conform to the regulatory standards of quality?
— Are all the ingredients safe and approved for their intended use in the UK and
other countries where sales are intended?
— If an ingredient is removed from the permitted list, is there an acceptable
alternative?
— Should time be allocated for regulatory clearance of an ingredient?
— Will the product contribute substantially to the diet?
— Is the product designed to be a replacement or alternative to a natural food, and
should it be nutritionally equivalent to the natural food it would simulate?

If nutrition claims (see section below) are desired or intended, further questions are
raised such as:

— Do the ingredients used support the claims?

— Would a nutrition claim trigger off any other labelling requirement?
— How much processing and storage data is necessary to support on-the-shelf nutrition claims?
— What extra quality control will the new product need to support the claims?

On the wide public relations issues, further question may arise:

— Can the consumer use the product without creating a hazard in the home?
— Are the cooking instructions adequate to ensure safety and product acceptability?
— Will the manufacturing process or packaging have any environmental impact?
— Are the ingredients perceived by consumers to be good or bad for you?
— How do misconceptions about some ingredients and environmental issues become imprinted in the consumer's mind?

From these sorts of questions, it is apparent that changes which influence the development of new products will come thick and fast in the next few years. Some of them will be completely unpredictable and the rewards will go to those companies that respond quickly and flexibly to the existing trends.

ATTITUDE OF THE CONSUMER TO MANUFACTURED FOODS

Total annual food consumption in the UK is virtually static and, therefore, it is changes in consumers' eating habits which influence the industry as a whole. Although food habits tend to be fairly stable, they can also be faddish and irrational, so that a decision to buy or eat a food may have different significance for different people on different occasions. The food scientists' view of health risks from food is given in Table 10.5 and this order of priority may vary considerably from the consumers perception.

Table 10.5 — The scientific assessment of risks from food

- Hazards of microbiological origin
- Nutritional hazards
- Environmental contaminants
- Natural food toxins
- Residues of agrochemicals
- Direct and indirect food additives

The consumer's awareness and quality expectations of a food product may be strongly influenced by a company's marketing and advertisements and by the kind of display and offers in the trade. All these activities are designed to initiate buying, but they have little effect upon the consumer's experience of the product in the home, or his/her decisions — based on satisfaction or disappointment — to buy again or stop buying. Assuming a new product does sell, then it is even more important to maintain a constant level of quality and to stimulate repeat purchases. The problem that the manufacturer faces is how to identify these characteristics of a food which are either liked or disliked by the consumer. The success or failure of an existing or new product lies in the hands of the consumer, and the texture, flavour and appearance are among the most important characteristics of foods and drinks because they are attributes which the consumer can readily perceive and assess (Plate 10.3). It is vital, therefore, to know in detail about the sensory aspects of products, and to be aware of the overall shifts and trends in sensory quality characteristics shown in Table 10.6.

Table 10.6 — Recent trends and changes in sensory attributes of food products

Dead/simple	$\longrightarrow$	live/complex
Preserved	$\longrightarrow$	fresh
Artificial	$\longrightarrow$	natural
Uniform	$\longrightarrow$	varied texture
Hot	$\longrightarrow$	cold
Heavy	$\longrightarrow$	light (calories)
Soggy	$\longrightarrow$	crunchy
Bland	$\longrightarrow$	spicy and clearly defined
Dominant	$\longrightarrow$	subtle
Sweet	$\longrightarrow$	savoury

Influence of dietary guidelines
National and international dietary guidelines reflect the general agreement of nutrition scientists that a more moderate diet, which avoids excessive amounts of fat, saturated fat, sugar, salt and alcohol, and contains more dietary fibre and starch, could help in reducing the risk of many of the degenerative diseases and chronic conditions from which most of us die eventually.

For example, in the UK, the COMA Report (DHSS, 1984), although pointing out the multifactorial nature of the degenerative diseases and the lack of absolute proof of the link between diet and these diseases, made the following recommendations to the food industry, which have been widely accepted:

(a) new product development in line with dietary guidelines
(b) more detailed food analysis and food composition data
(c) more nutrition information on packs

Manufacturers are aware of the need to adapt to changes in consumer eating habits and attitudes to the quality of food, and most companies are continually pursuing extensive research and development programmes to ensure that the existing products and new product developments match consumer demand. For example, consumer interest in the fibre content of foods has increased greatly in recent years. Unfortunately, publicity and speculation on the role of dietary fibre in the prevention of some diseases have run ahead of the available scientific facts. Nevertheless, the imagination of the consumer has been captured by the belief that fibre is a 'health-giving ingredient', and as a result, the

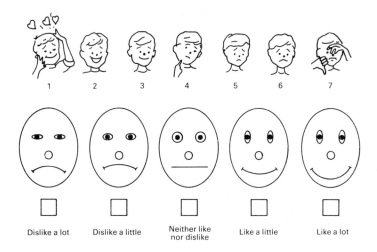

□	□	□	□	□
Dislike a lot	Dislike a little	Neither like nor dislike	Like a little	Like a lot

Plate 10.3 — Texture, flavour and appearance are among the most important characteristics of foods and drinks because they are attributes which the consumer can readily perceive and assess.

so-called 'dietary fibre' and 'muesli' markets are growing quickly. Almost all breakfast cereals seem to boast of added bran. Snacks, biscuits and breads containing fibre represent other avenues of product development, and in these the fibre component not only conveys several important functional and textural properties which can not only be advantageous in product manufacture, but can also be promoted as providing a nutritional benefit.

Another growth area is for yoghurts, and low-fat fruit-flavoured yoghurts in particular. To consumers, yoghurts are considered to be natural and healthy, and in some way to contribute to longevity. However, although many consumers associate low-fat yoghurts with slimming, the varieties which contain fruit and are sweetened with sugar are by no means low-calorie foods.

A further indication of the growing consumer interest in health and fitness is the market in low-calories and slimming foods. Low-calorie soups, salad creams and dressings, sweeteners, soft drinks, wines and beers, in addition to a vast range of slimming aids and calorie-controlled meals, are now widely available. It is estimated that two out of five people in the UK purchase low-calorie items on a regular basis.

Changes in Consumption Patterns
Today, consumers are trading up to higher quality, more complex, fresher, more 'natural' and better tasting foods. For example, some of the major trends in food consumption, which directly influence the food industry, are an increase in the consumption of convenience, frozen and chilled foods. There is a continuing decline in the popularity of canned goods, a steady move away from sugar, whole milk and butter, red meats, bacon,

sausages, eggs and salt. At the same time, there is increased consumption of brown, wholemeal and speciality breads at the expense of white bread, and increases in consumption of yoghurt, fresh leafy salads, soft fruits, vegetables, salad oils and a wide range of snack foods such as crisps, nuts and dried fruits. The trend towards 'healthy' eating is now well established; but despite this, there is a strongly developing 'indulgent' factor, which has created a growth in markets for luxury and exotic food products.

Demographic changes
In the UK, within a stable total population, the ages and structure of the population will have major implications for product development. There is a significant decline in the number of young adults, a substantially increasing number of elderly and affluent consumers, a significant increase in the family foundation group (the post-war 'baby boomers') and an increasing number of households with fewer people in them. It is, therefore, relatively easy to predict that single servings and foods in special, convenient, easy-to-open packaging will be purchased with increasing frequency.

Shopping
The buying strength of the large retail multiples and the concentration of shopping into fewer, larger, out-of-town stores already has had enormous impact on food purchases. The development of sophisticated computer information systems to track individual product performance, analyse sales and streamline stocking and inventory controls has also been important in strengthening the control of the retailer on the food chain. As well as this, retailers have promoted nutrition as a major selling theme at the point of purchase by the use of healthy eating brochures and the like. One aspect of the concentration of food retailing which has had little attention is that those customers without personal transport and those who are elderly or infirm or poor may find difficulties in obtaining adequate supplies of food because of the sheer physical difficulties in carrying groceries home. Hence, there may be many opportunities for a revival of smaller local shops and for speedy home-delivery systems.

Revolution in the home
Today, the kitchen is more often than not the focal point of the household. Electronic technology, labour-saving devices, and perhaps most newsworthy — the microwave oven — all influence product development. The microwave oven is the second most popular piece of electrical equipment to the electric kettle and over 40 per cent of all households in the UK have one. Microwave ovens save time, and used properly, can preserve nutrients, but learning to use one is like learning to cook all over again. Many food manufacturers are now providing the 'do's' and 'don'ts' instructions on labels to inform consumers about product safety, quality and optimal nutritional value.

Worries about health and food
A continuous survey carried out since September 1986 in the UK has indicated that far

Table 10.7 —Consumer attitudes towards food ingredients considered very bad or quite bad, together with their perceived views on the content of a 'healthy' food. (% of respondents agreeing with statement)

Very bad/quite bad	%	Very good	%
Fats	86	Vitamins	49
Additives	81	Fibre	40
Sugar	78	Protein	39
Colourings	74	Low in fat	25
Cholesterol	73	Freshness	25
Salt	72	Iron	19
Preservatives	68	Low in sugar	18
E numbers	66	Few additives	18
Flavourings	58		
Artificial sweeteners	47		

Data from Jones Rhodes Associates, 1988.

more people today are concerned about food and their health than in the past (see Table 10.7). Fats, additives, sugar, cholesterol, salt, colourings, preservatives, E numbers, flavourings and artificial sweeteners are the major food components described by respondents as 'very bad' or 'quite bad'. For comparison, the attributes of a healthy food include vitamins, fibre, protein, low fat, freshness, iron, low sugar and absence of certain food additives. The media have done much to stimulate consumer interest in nutrition, but sometimes overenthusiasm for good 'copy' has led to a certain degree of misinformation being disseminated to the public.

More and more advertising campaigns contain information about food safety and nutrition and highlight quality attributes which relate specifically to consumer concerns about diet, safety and health. In addition, many manufacturers have demonstrated that good nutrition and 'healthier' lifestyle can sell food products.

Consumers whose interest in nutrition has been awakened will want sound, authoratative information to be able to assess the nutritional value of the foods they consume, and they will look increasingly to the food label to supply this information. Furthermore, the success of any kind of dietary modifications, whether for the individual or as a public health measure, depends on the buying public having a better understanding of nutrition.

Communicating nutrition and healthy eating

Food labelling and, in particular, the use of nutrition and health claims are potentially the most significant food policy issues. However, by placing any information on to a package label, manufacturers and retailers engage merely in printing - nothing more. To be effective, any system of labelling should act as the cornerstone of an education policy, and the basic objective should be a system which is:

— consumer-orientated and meaningful
— helpful at the point of purchase

—suitable for people to select balanced diets or to follow recommended diets
— applicable to a wide range of foods.

In addition, any effort to develop and control claims should:

— permit fair trade and competition (nationally and internationally);
— restrict the use of spurious claims;
— eliminate emphasis on nutritional qualities of only marginal importance, which give a completely erroneous impression of the food and its use.

Nutrition labelling, therefore, can provide the crucial basic nutrition information for wise choices and decision making. If the information is up-to-date, accurate, easy to read and in a consistent format, it can provide essential facts. But this provision of data on labels is only a starting point, and not a substitute for more wide-ranging education.

Nutritional and compositional databases

Technical accuracy and compliance with specific legal requirements need a comprehensive food composition data system. Today, the maintenance of records of compositional standards and nutrition profiles is an awesome task. To ensure that all on-pack statements and claims can be substantiated requires specialist assessment and collation of data on raw materials, semi-processed materials and finished products, good control and unique numbering of recipes, careful checking of analytical work, scrutiny of calculations and specialist input of information into the database. Many of the larger companies now have their own nutritional and compositional databases. The databases can provide:

Nutrition information for:

    Declaration on pack
    Sales Brochures
    Tenders/contracts
    Dietary information sheets
    Nutrition claims
    Private label specification

Product information for:

    Legal compliance
    Claims on pack and in advertising
    Private label specifications
    Consumer enquiries
    Government enquiries
    Media enquiries
    Export tariff refunds

Food intolerance databases:
    'Free from' and 'contains' lists, such as those established by the Leatherhead Food

Research Association in collaboration with the British Dietetic Association and the food manufacturing industry.

The Leatherhead Food Intolerance Databank comprises well over 400 manufactured foods. It embraces foods which are 'free from' at least one of the 'top ten' food components most commonly associated with food intolerance. The 'top ten' list was compiled by clinical experts to reflect practical experience and includes milk and milk derivatives, soya and soya derivatives, cocoa, DHA and BHT, sulphur dioxide, benzoate, glutamate and azo colours.

Given the importance of nutrition labelling, it is essential to have a harmonized format in this country and throughout Europe. It is also especially necessary to find ways which can be used in the multilingual context of the 1992 European market without frontiers; to ensure that the amount, quality and availability of food composition data are properly coordinated; to emphasize the need and agreement for common methods of analyses internationally; and to ensure expression of information is compatible. Here lies a real opportunity for governments and the food industry to collaborate to develop and expand existing compositional databases.

NUTRITION AND FOOD LAW

The past few years have seen a marked increase in technical food legislation, primarily as a result of our membership of the EC, but also as a result of increasing interest in the safety, composition and nutritional value of foods by the regulatory agencies, consumers, media and the food industry. In England and Wales, the Food Act 1984 lays down the basic provisions of food law covering the composition, labelling and wholesomeness of food. There are equivalent provisions in Scotland and Northern Ireland. Other legal requirements are governed by the Food Labelling Regulations, the Weights and Measures Act, the Trade Descriptions Act. the Food, and Environment Protection Act and more recently, the Consumer Protection Act. These Acts are supplemented by specific regulations and Orders, Codes of Practice and Advice Notes. In total, there are 10 Acts of Parliament and over 175 Statutory Instruments controlling all aspects of food production, composition, labelling, hygiene and marketing, ranging from the farm gate to liability from any injury concerned.

This statutory framework and the provisions of the law must all be used together if food products are to be labelled correctly. Table 10.8 shows the various legislative measures in the UK involving labelling. Legal liability may arise with respect to both mandatory information and voluntary information, and hence all statements must be correct, and all claims must be capable of being substantiated under existing law. Table 10.9 shows the areas in which a criminal offence may be committed. Compliance with the details of regulations and codes of practice is not only a necessity but it contributes materially and positively to the production of safe, competitive, quality food products. Table 10.10 shows those nutritional claims which are regulated by the Food Labelling Regulations (1984). Tables 10.11 and 10.12 summarize the detailed conditions for making claims about vitamins. Identical conditions exist for claims for minerals. Table 10.3 shows those vitamins and minerals in respect of which claims may be made under the Food Labelling Regulations 1984.

Table 10.8 — Food labelling controls

• General labelling requirements are imposed by the Food Act, the Trade Descriptions Acts, the Weights and Measures Act and, in particular, by the Food Labelling Regulations.

• These are supplemented by Specific Product Sector Regulations which control Reserved Descriptions, Compositional Standards and, in some instances, even the layout of specified declarations and the form of words to be used.

• This statutory framework is further supplemented by Codes of Practice, Advice Notes and Court Decisions clarifying the provisions of the law.

   ALL THE ABOVE MUST BE READ TOGETHER IF PRODUCTS ARE TO BE LABELLED CORRECTLY

• Legal liability may arise in respect of both *mandatory* and *voluntary* information.

   ALL STATEMENTS MUST THEREFORE BE CORRECT AND ALL CLAIMS CAPABLE OF BEING SUBSTANTIATED

Mandatory information	Voluntary information
Name/true description	Price mark
Minimum durability (unless exempt)	e mark
Weight mark (unless exempt)	Nutrition labelling
Ingredients list	Additive/'free from' claims/
Storage conditions	'naturalness'
Name and address etc.	Royal warrants
% declarations: special emphasis	'Special emphasis'
specific products	Honest pictorials
True 'presentation'	Nutritional claims
Origin (if necessary)	controlled by labelling
	regulations
	Special offers
	Use of 'PLUS' words — e.g.
	healthy, rich, creamy
	original etc.

Additional Nutrition Claims

Within the legal context mentioned above and with the current interest in nutrition, 'healthy' eating, food additives and 'naturalness', the food industry has been stimulated to develop a remarkable number of products claiming nutritional benefits such as less fat, less sugar, less salt, enriched with fibre, vitamins, minerals, calcium, free from additives etc. In a few cases, these claims have implied improvements in health which cannot be fully substantiated, and there has been a huge increase in 'negative' and 'comparative' claims (see below) which can lead to technical and legal difficulties as well as confusion. Reputable food manufacturers share the concerns, held by MAFF and consumer organizations, that different sectors of the food industry have taken different approaches to respond to customer demands for more information about the foods we eat, and it is recognized that there is a need for a consistent policy across the whole spectrum of products to cover such aspects as technical terminology and nutrition claims on labels in advertising.

Labelling policies, marketing and promotional strategies should be developed that will enable customers to make informed choices and to enjoy the benefits of all that modern food manufacturing technology can provide. Indeed, the developments of many of the so-called healthy products have required considerable technological skills as well as large commercial investments.

Recently, the Food Advisory Committee (FAC), has recommended that new legislative controls are necessary to regulate the use of comparative claims flashed on food labels, and used in advertising, including statements about the 'high', 'low' and 'reduced' levels of certain components such as fat, sugar, sodium and fibre. The Ministry of Agriculture, Fisheries and Food (MAFF) has indicated its intention to recommend legislation for these types of claims. Its recommendations are summarized in Appendix 1. MAFF has published the FAC proposals not only as an advance indication for the UK food industry but also as a basis for negotiation, should the European Commission step in and propose controls on nutrition claims of this type. The FAC proposals may provide a new framework for the harmonization of these types of claims throughout the Community. All the claims trigger off the compulsory declaration of the MAFF Category II (Big 8) format as shown in Table 10.14.

Table 10.9 — Criminal offences

Under the Food Act:

● Fasely describe food
● Label/advertise food misleadingly as to nature, substance or quality

Under the Trade Descriptions Act:

● Apply a false trade description to any goods

Table 10.10 — Regulated nutritional claims in the United Kingdom

---

Dietetic
Baby/Infant
Diabetic
Slimming
Medicinal
Protein
Vitamin
Mineral
Polyunsaturates
Cholesterol
Energy

Table 10.11 — The types of, and conditions for, vitamin claims on food labels when the claims are confined to named vitamins

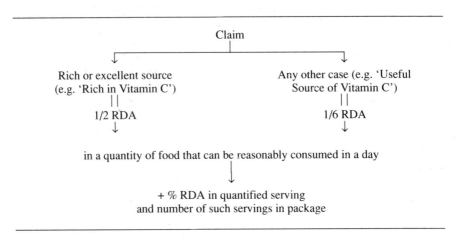

RDA, Recommended Daily Amounts
Conditions for minerals are the same as above

Table 10.12 — The types of, and conditions for, vitamin claims on food labels when the claims are not confined to named vitamins

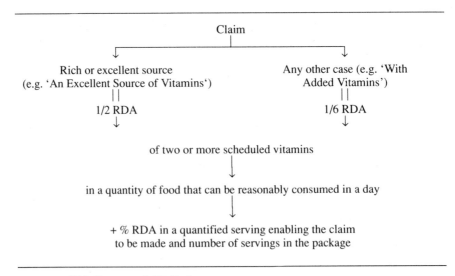

RDA, Recommended Daily Amounts
Conditions for minerals are the same as above

Appendix 1

Food Advisory Committee Recommendations (1989) for nutrition claims in food labelling and advertising

Source: MAFF (1989) Food Advisory Committee. *Proposals on the use of nutrition claims in the labelling and advertising of food*. HMSO, London.

FAT, SUGAR, SODIUM

Claims	Conditions
Reduced	
Reduced fat or saturates Reduced sugar§ or sugars§ Reduced salt or sodium	At least 25% reduction compared with a similar food typical of those for which no claim is made
No added	
No added sugars No added sugars Unsweetened[IP]	No mono- or disaccharides or food composed mainly of these sugars should have been added to the food or to any of its ingredients
No added salt No added sodium	No sodium chloride or other salts of sodium should have been added to the food or to any of its ingredients

Low	**Max/100 g food wt**	**AND**	**Max/Normal serving* wt**
Low fat‡ Low in saturates‡	Total fat 5 g/100g Total saturates 3 g/100g		Total fat 5 g Total saturates 3 g
Low in sugar‡ Low in sugars‡	Total sugars 5 g/100g		Total sugars 5 g
Low in salt‡ Low in sodium‡	Total sodium 40 mg/100g		Total sodium 40 mg

Free			
Fat free	Total fat 0.15 g/100g		NR
Saturates free	Total saturates 0.1 g/100g		NR
Sugar free	Total sugars 0.2 g/100g		NR
Sugars free			
Salt free	Total sodium 5 mg/100g		NR
Sodium free			

FIBRE

Claims	**Conditions**
Source of fibre†	Total fibre at least 3g/100g food *or* 3g/'reasonable daily intake'
Higher fibre More fibre Increased fibre	At least 25% increase compared with a similar food typical of those for which no claim is made, AND total fibre at least 3g/100g food *or* 3g/'reasonable daily intake'
High in fibre‡ † Rich in fibre‡ †	Total fibre at least 6g/100g food *or* 6g/'reasonable daily intake'

NB: ALL OF THE ABOVE CLAIMS WOULD REQUIRE CATEGORY III DECLARATION.

*   Where normal serving is less than 50g or ml or more than 150g, Category III declaration required for a given specified serving.

†   Where claim is based on reasonable daily intake or serving, Category III declaration required for a given specified serving. Fibre calculated as non-starch polysaccharides.

Where the claim appears in advertising, claim must be substantiated in the advertisement.

‡   If food naturally low in fat, claim 'A low fat food' required
    If food naturally low in saturates, claim 'A low saturates food' required
    If food naturally low in sugars, claim 'A low sugar food' required.
    If food naturally low in sodium, claim 'A low salt/sodium food' required
    If food naturally high in fibre, claim 'A high fibre food' required.
§   Not applicable to Jams and Similar Products Reg. 1981 (as amnd)
IP Not applicable to provisions in Condensed Milk & Dried Milk Regs. 1977 (as amnd).

Where food is concentrated or dehydrated and is intended to be reconstituted by the addition of water or other substances, the conditions above apply to the food when reconstituted as directed.

NR No recommendation

Appendix 2

Food Advisory Committee Guidelines (1989) on 'natural claims'[†] in the labelling, advertising and presentation of food

ALLOWED, BUT CONDITIONAL

(a) **Simple traditional foods:**

No additions, and minimal processing sufficient to render them suitable for human consumption.

(b) **Ingredients:**

As (a) above, and from recognized food sources.

(c) **Flavourings/additives:**

From recognized food sources using either physical processes *or* traditional food preparation processes. Flavouring to be *wholly* from named food source.

(d) **Compound foods not regarded as natural:**

Can claim 'made from natural ingredients' only if all ingredients comply with (b) and (c) above.

(e) **Natural flavour, taste or colour:**

Only if complying with (a) or (b) above.

(f) **'Natural' meaning just plain or unflavoured:**

Only if complying with (a) or (b) above.

(g) **Brand or fancy names etc:**
Not to include/reflect/imply naturalness unless complies with (a) or (d) above.

NOT ALLOWED

Natural goodness
Naturally better   and all similar
Nature's way

NB: The same principles apply to words similar to 'natural' such as 'real', 'genuine', 'pure' *when they are used in place of 'natural' in such a way as to imply similar benefits to consumers.*

†Source: MAFF (1989) Food Advisory Committee. *Guidelines on the use of natural and similar terms in the labelling, advertising and presentation of foods.* HMSO, London.

Appendix 3

Food Advisory Committee Guidelines (1989) on 'negative claims'† in the labelling, advertising and presentation of food

FAC considers that 'negative claims', which do not use the term 'natural' or its derivatives but the effect of which is to imply naturalness to the consumer, are potentially misleading and confusing.

ALLOWED, BUT CONDITIONAL

'Free from X' or 'No X':
Only if all similar foods *contain X*, where X is a class or category of additive, e.g. if a Fruit Drink contains no preservative but other brands do, then the product can claim 'free from preservatives'.

AND

'No artificial X' or 'Free from artificial X':
Only if product free from X and other artificial additives, and no undue emphasis is made by the claim, where X is an artificial or non-natural additive, e.g. if a product has *no* artificial colour and contains *no* other artificial additives, then can claim 'no artificial colours' (no undue emphasis).

AND

'Free from X' or 'No X':
Only if product contains no other additives or ingredients having broadly similar

effect as *X*, where *X* is a category of additive, e.g. (a) if a product contains no stabilizers but does contain modified starch, *cannot* claim it is 'free from stabilizers'; (b) if a product contains *no* tartrazine colour, but *does* contain sunset yellow, a tartrazine free claim *cannot* be made.

NB: Where it is assumed that '**Free from** *X*' does *not* imply 'naturalness' to the consumer, FAC accepts that this may provide accurate and beneficial information for the consumer, where *X* is a *particular* additive.

† Source: MAFF (1989) Food Advisory Committee. *Guidelines on the use of natural and similar terms in the labelling, advertising and presentation of food.* HMSO, London.

Index